MIND, MUSCLE, & MOTION

YOUR ULTIMATE FITNESS BLUEPRINT

Let's embark on a fitness journey as we explore the path to a healthier, stronger you.

By
Saheeb Dadan

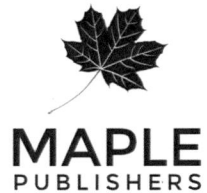

MAPLE
PUBLISHERS

MIND, MUSCLE, & MOTION

Author: Saheeb Dadan

Copyright © Saheeb Dadan (2024)

The right of Saheeb Dadan to be identified as author of this work has been asserted by the author in accordance with section 77 and 78 of the Copyright, Designs and Patents Act 1988.

First Published in 2024

ISBN 978-1-83538-210-3 (Paperback)
　　　978-1-83538-211-0 (Hardback)
　　　978-1-83538-212-7 (E-Book)

Book Layout by:
　　　White Magic Studios
　　　www.whitemagicstudios.co.uk

Published by:
　　　Maple Publishers
　　　Fairbourne Drive, Atterbury,
　　　Milton Keynes,
　　　MK10 9RG, UK
　　　www.maplepublishers.com

A CIP catalogue record for this title is available from the British Library.

All rights reserved. No part of this book may be reproduced or translated by any form or by any means, electronic or mechanical, including photocopying, recording or by any information storage and retrieval system without written permission from the author.

The views expressed in this work are solely those of the author and do not necessarily reflect the views of the publisher, and the publisher hereby disclaims any responsibility for them.

"I'm not the strongest, I'm not the biggest, but I'm damn sure the toughest." – **Ronnie Coleman**

"I hated every minute of training, but I said, 'Don't quit, suffer now and live the rest of your life as a champion.'" – **Muhammad Ali**

"The only way to grow is to challenge yourself." – **Lou Ferrigno**

"A Fitness Dynamo: A Personal Journey into Fitness, Nutrition and the benefits of becoming an Athlete".

Saheeb Dadan

Contents

Introduction – The Awakening 5

Chapter 1 – Setting the Foundation 7

Chapter 2 – The Sweat Equity 10

Chapter 3 – Nutrition Nourishment 14

Chapter 4 – Has Ashwagandha gained significant attention in Bodybuilding? 31

Chapter 5 – The Plateau and Perseverance 34

Chapter 6 – The Myths of Fitness & Bodybuilding. 37

Chapter 7 – How do the Myths in Fitness impact you as an Athlete? 40

Chapter 8 – What is the secret behind a Summer body? 42

Chapter 9 – How do Cheat Meals impact your fitness journey? 46

Chapter 10 – Is Beast mode all about Ego? 49

Chapter 11 – Training Routine for Beginners, Intermediaries and Advanced. 53

Chapter 12 – My Ultimate Abs Workout routine. 63

Chapter 13 – Are supplements more important than food in bodybuilding? 68

Chapter 14 – The basics of diet plan. 71

Chapter 15 – The Get-Ripped Foods. 80

Chapter 16 – The 8 golden rules to stay Ripped the whole year. 84

Chapter 17 – Why is it so important to train with like-minded people? (Community & Camaraderie) 90

Chapter 18 – The Blue Gym of Superheroes. 96

Chapter 19 – Should you have a personal Trainer or Mentor? 118

Chapter 20 – The Finish Line and Beyond. 121

Acknowledgement 124

Introduction

The Awakening

"My fitness journey continues. The pages of my journal filled with new goals: A pull-up, A push-up, and maybe even a handstand. But one thing remains constant, the power of writing it down. So, grab your pen, open your heart, and let your fitness journey unfold, one step, one rep, one word at a time".

In the quiet of my living room, I sat on the couch, staring at the TV screen. The latest reality show blared, and I realized something: I was a spectator in my own life. My body had become a shapeless lump, and my energy levels were plummeting. It was time for a change. A change of a lifetime, a change of fitness that was about to shape my body from a 0 to a 100. A journey to self-transformation. From sedentary to striving, breaking the chains in the cocoon of comfort, I once resided, a couch-potato, content with inertia. But life nudged me awake. It whispered, "Move!" And so, I did. I stepped into the gym, unsure and trembling. Each treadmill stride became a declaration: "I am more than my sedentary self."

The notes of resilience rang in my ears, As the weights clanged and the elliptical hummed, I discovered a symphony within. Sweat dripped, but so did excuses. The rhythm of my breath synced with the grind of the machines. I realized that fitness wasn't just about muscles; it was about resilience, the ability to push beyond limits.

I started having mirror conversations, reflections of change the gym mirror became my confidante. It didn't lie. It reflected my sweat-soaked determination, my flushed cheeks, and the fire in my eyes. With each bicep curl, I whispered affirmations: "I am strong. I am capable." And slowly, the reflection transformed, a metamorphosis fuelled by sweat equity.

The Awakening

The power of consistency grew within me, I made consistency my silent companion, it held my hand. It taught me that progress isn't a sprint; it's a marathon. Day after day, I returned, to the treadmill, the dumbbells, the mat, all witnesses to my commitment. And in that repetition, I found growth. Not just physical, but soul deep.

My journal held my journey, the early doubts, the sore muscles, and the moments of sheer determination. But it also held my transformation, the stronger the body, the clearer the mind, and the newfound confidence.

Beyond the Gym Walls

Life Lessons:

Fitness seeped beyond the gym walls. It infused my choices, my relationships, my purpose. I learned:

1. **Self-Discipline**: The gym clock doesn't wait; neither should I.
2. **Resilience**: Muscles ache, but they rebuild stronger.
3. **Self-Love**: Sweat isn't a sign of weakness; it's a badge of effort.
4. **Community**: High-fives from fellow warriors, proof that we're in this together.

The awakening of fitness isn't about six-pack abs or marathon medals. It's about unravelling layers, discovering grit, and rewriting narratives. So, dear reader, lace up your sneakers. Let the weights sing their song. Your awakening awaits, a symphony of sweat, strength, and self-discovery.

You are more than flesh and bone; you are resilience personified.

Remember, you're not alone. We're all on this journey together.

Chapter 1
Setting the Foundation

Setting a Strong Foundation in the Gym: Your Blueprint for Success

Congratulations on taking the first step toward a healthier, stronger you! Whether you're a gym newbie or returning after a hiatus, building a solid foundation is crucial. In this book, we'll explore essential principles, practical tips, and actionable steps to set you up for long-term fitness success.

Grab a pen and a blank notebook. This would be your fitness journal—a record of sweat, sore muscles, and triumphs. Write down your goals: lose weight, gain strength, and run 5K. Each day, log your workouts, meals, and feelings. The act of writing makes it real.

Embrace the New Environment

The Gym Landscape

- **Overcoming Intimidation**: The gym can feel overwhelming, especially with seasoned lifters grunting and machines galore. Remember, everyone starts somewhere. You belong here too!
- **Knowledge Is Power**: Rather than stressing about the "perfect" routine, focus on learning. Absorb information, observe, and ask questions. With knowledge, you craft your fitness symphony. Knowledge empowers you to optimize power.

Speak the Language

- **Exercise Names**: Learning the names of exercises serves multiple purposes:

- **Research**: When Google fails you, knowing the exercise names helps you find proper form and variations.
- **Communication**: Chat with trainers or fellow gym-goers confidently.
- **Tracking**: Efficiently log your workouts.

Gym Etiquette

Respect the Space

- **Boundaries**: Be mindful of others' personal space.
- **Courtesy**: Treat trainers and fellow gym enthusiasts with kindness.
- **Mirror Manners**: Don't block someone's view—especially near the mirrors.
- **Hygiene**: Wear deodorant, wipe down equipment, and carry a towel.

Warm-Up Rituals

Why Warm Up Matters

- **Physical Prep**: A proper warm-up primes your body for exercise.
- **Injury Prevention**: Stretching reduces stiffness and minimizes injury risk.
- **Blood Flow Boost**: Get that blood pumping!

Foundational Exercises

Master the Basics

- **Squat**: The king of compound movements. Learn proper form and variations.
- **Deadlift**: Builds overall strength. Nail your technique.
- **Push-Ups**: Simple yet effective for chest, shoulders, and triceps.
- **Pull-Ups**: Develop upper body strength.

Consistency and Patience

Slow and Steady Wins
- **Consistency**: Show up regularly. Progress accumulates over time.
- **Celebrate Small Wins**: Each rep, each session counts.
- **Mindset**: Trust the process. Results will follow.

Conclusion

Remember, Rome wasn't built in a day, and neither is your fitness journey. Lay a strong foundation, stay curious, and enjoy the process. You're on your way to becoming a gym dynamo!

Chapter 2

The Sweat Equity

The gym became my second home. I sweated through cardio sessions, lifted weights, and tried yoga for the first time. My journal filled with numbers—reps, miles, and calories burned. But it wasn't just about the physical fitness. I journaled about my mental victories too—the days I pushed through fatigue or conquered self-doubt.

Sweat Equity in the Gym: Unlocking Your Fitness Potential

Welcome to the world of sweat equity! In this book, we'll delve into the concept of sweat equity as it relates to your fitness journey. Whether you're a seasoned gym-goer or a newbie stepping onto the treadmill for the first time, understanding and harnessing the power of sweat can transform your workouts.

What Is Sweat Equity?

The Sweat Equation

Sweat equity is the currency of effort you invest during your workouts. It's not just about the physical perspiration; it's about the mental and emotional commitment too. Think of it as a balance sheet: on one side, you have the calories burned, muscles engaged, and heart rate elevated; on the other, you gain strength, endurance, and a sense of accomplishment.

The Science Behind Sweat

Why Do We Sweat?
- **Thermoregulation**: Sweating helps regulate body temperature. As you exercise, your internal furnace cranks up, and sweat acts as the cooling system.

- **Detoxification**: Sweat carries away toxins and impurities, leaving you feeling refreshed.
- **Endorphin Release**: Ever heard of a "runner's high"? Sweat triggers the release of endorphins, those magical mood-boosting chemicals.

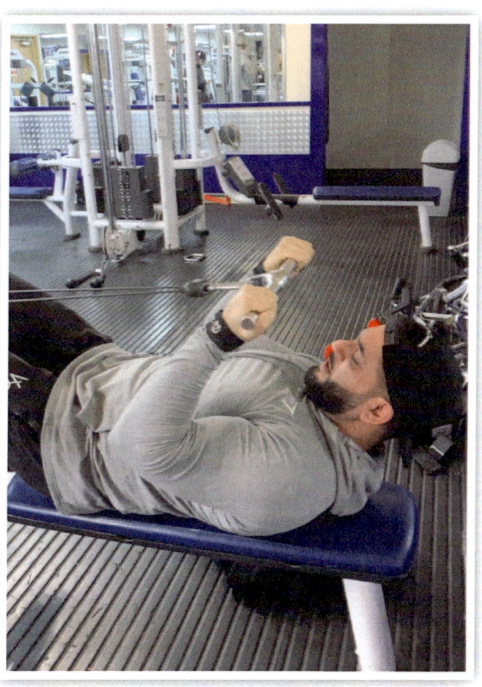

Types of Sweat Equity

1. Cardiovascular Sweat
   - **Treadmill Troopers**: Running, cycling, and dancing—anything that gets your heart pumping.
   - **HIIT Heroes**: High-Intensity Interval Training (HIIT) sessions that leave you breathless and drenched.
2. Strength Sweat
   - **Iron Warriors**: Weightlifting, resistance training, and body weight exercises.
   - **Yoga Yodas**: Yes, even in yoga, you're sweating out toxins and building strength.

The Sweat Equity

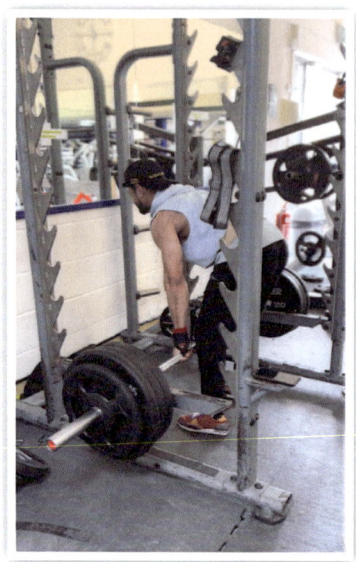

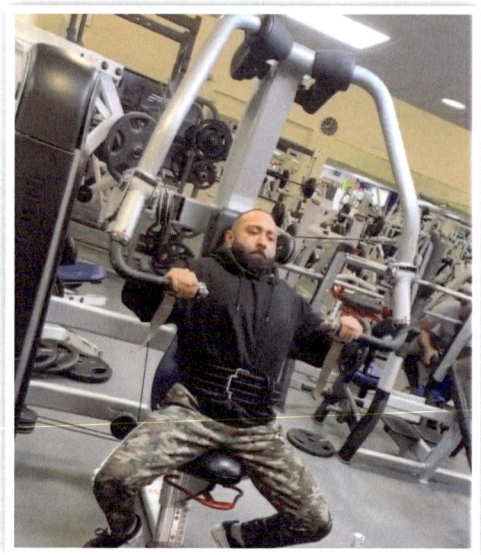

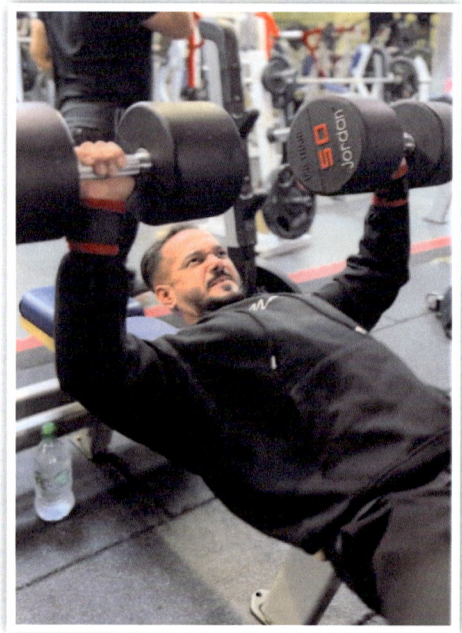

Maximizing Your Sweat Investment

1. Hydration Matters
    - **Drink Up**: Proper hydration ensures efficient sweating. Aim for at least 8 glasses of water a day.

- **Electrolytes**: Replenish those lost salts with electrolyte-rich drinks.

2. Nutrition for Sweat Warriors
    - **Fuel Your Fire**: Balanced meals with protein, carbs, and healthy fats keep your sweat engine running.
    - **Pre-Workout Snacks**: Grab a banana (yes, the same one we measured Everest with!) or some almonds.

3. Embrace the Drip
    - **Celebrate Sweat**: It's proof that you're pushing your limits.
    - **Visualize Your Goals**: Imagine your dream physique as you drip onto the gym floor.

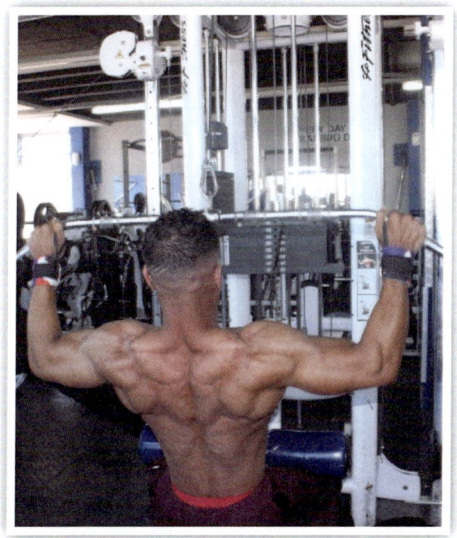

Conclusion

Sweat equity isn't just about calories burned; it's about the transformation that happens within. So, lace up those sneakers, grab a towel, and step into the gym. Your sweat is your investment—watch it pay dividends in strength, health, and confidence.

Remember: **Sweat today, shine tomorrow!**

Chapter 3

Nutrition Nourishment

Fuelling Your Mind, Muscle and Soul

My kitchen transformed. I swapped chips for carrot sticks, soda for water, and fast food for homemade meals. My journal tracked my food choices, revealing patterns and pitfalls. I learned that nutrition was the fuel for my fitness journey. And yes, I celebrated the occasional indulgence too—because balance matters.

In the symphony of life, nutrition plays a pivotal role—a harmonious blend of science, sustenance, and self-care. Welcome to *Nutrition Nourishment*, where we explore the art of nourishing not just our bodies but our entire being.

The Essence of Nourishment

Beyond Calories

Nutrition—A word often reduced to calorie counting and food labels. But it's more profound. It's about **nourishing**—providing our cells, tissues, and spirit with the raw materials they crave. Let's dive into the heart of nourishment.

The Nutrient Symphony

Vitamins, Minerals, and More

Our bodies are orchestras, and nutrients are the notes. From vitamin C's bright crescendo to iron's steady bassline, each nutrient contributes to our vitality. We'll explore the dance of vitamins, the rhythm of minerals, and the harmony of proteins.

A - Vitamins: These tiny conductors orchestrate cellular processes. In the intricate tapestry of nutrition, vitamins are the vibrant threads that weave our well-being. Welcome to *Vitamins: Unravelling Their Mysteries and Impact on Health*, where we explore these micronutrients beyond their mere chemical structures.

A Century of Discovery

From Beriberi to Biochemistry

Vitamins emerged from the shadows a mere century ago, altering the course of human health. We'll delve into their fascinating history—their role in preventing and curing diseases that once haunted us.

The Alphabet of Health

Meet the Players

1. **Vitamin A**: The guardian of vision and immune function.
2. **Vitamin C**: The antioxidant maestro, defending against free radicals.
3. **Vitamin D**: Sun-kissed and bone-friendly.
4. **Vitamin K**: Covertly orchestrating blood clotting.

Beyond the Pill Bottle

Food as Medicine

While supplements beckon from pharmacy shelves, let's not forget their natural abode—our plates. We'll explore vitamin-rich foods—their flavours, colours, and synergy with other nutrients.

The Sunshine Vitamin and More

Vitamin D's Secrets

1. **Sunlight Synthesis**: Our skin's magical conversion.
2. **Immune Boost**: Beyond bones, vitamin D fortifies our defences.
3. **Deficiency Dilemmas**: From rickets to mood swings.

Navigating the Hype

Miracle or Myth?

1. **Antioxidant Obsession**: Separating fact from fad.
2. **Supplement Saga**: The Wild West of overpromising.
3. **Balance and Bioavailability**: Quality matters.

Vitamin it's a journey through science, history, and platefuls of vitality. So, raise your glass of orange juice, savour those leafy greens, and remember: **In this alphabet soup of health, each vitamin whispers its unique story.**

B - Minerals: Minerals are treasure of earth's crust. The silent architects of bone strength and nerve function. In the bustling gymnasiums and on the open trails, minerals play a silent yet profound role in our fitness journey. Welcome to *Minerals in Fitness: Unleashing the Power of Earth's Hidden Gems*, where we dig deep into these micronutrients and their impact on our physical prowess.

The Unsung Heroes

Minerals are the unsung heroes behind the scenes, ensuring our bodies function optimally. These inorganic elements—forged in the fiery depths of the Earth—hold the keys to our vitality. Let's explore their significance:

1. **Calcium:** Not just for bones; it's the conductor of muscle contractions, ensuring smooth movements during workouts. Calcium is essential for the development, health, and continued maintenance of **strong bones**. It contributes to bone density and helps prevent conditions like **osteoporosis**, especially 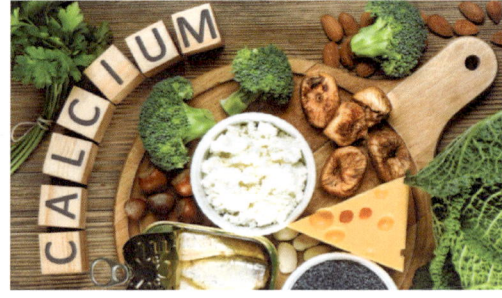 in women beyond menopause. Adequate calcium levels are

necessary for **muscle function**. When a muscle is stimulated, calcium is released, allowing the muscle to contract. Conversely, when calcium is pumped out of the muscle, it relaxes. This balance is crucial for smooth muscle movement during exercise.

Recommended Dietary Allowance (RDA) of Calcium (in milligrams):

1. **0–6 months**: 200 mg
2. **7–12 months**: 260 mg
3. **1–3 years**: 700 mg
4. **4–8 years**: 1,000 mg
5. **9–13 years**: 1,300 mg
6. **14–18 years**: 1,300 mg
7. **19–50 years**: 1,000 mg
8. **51–70 years**: 1,000 mg (males and females)
9. **70+ years**: 1,200 mg (males and females)

2. **Magnesium:** The relaxation mineral—essential for muscle recovery and preventing cramps. Magnesium contributes to bone density and may help prevent conditions like **osteoporosis**. It's essential for maintaining strong bones. Higher magnesium intake is linked to a **lower risk of heart disease**. It helps regulate blood pressure and supports cardiovascular health. Magnesium may enhance exercise performance. It helps transport blood sugar into muscles and clears lactate, which can cause fatigue during physical activity. Some studies suggest that magnesium supplements benefit muscle recovery and protect against muscle damage after strenuous 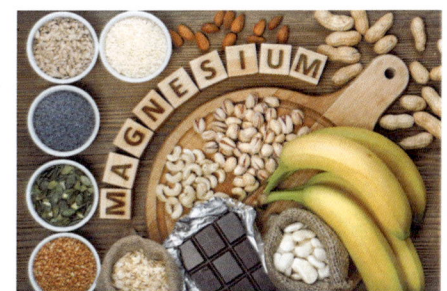 exercise. It also supports in Energy creation, Gene Maintenance, Muscle movements, and nervous system regulations.

3. **Iron:** The oxygen carrier, fuelling our cells during intense exercise. **Iron** is a vital mineral with numerous benefits for overall health. Iron is crucial for the production of **haemoglobin**, a protein in red blood cells (RBCs). Haemoglobin binds to oxygen, allowing RBCs to transport oxygen from the lungs to various tissues throughout 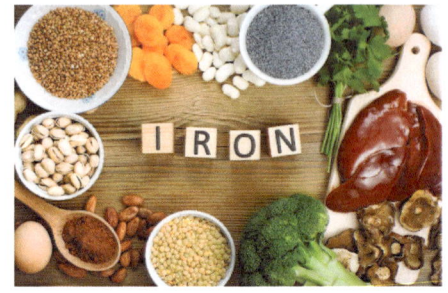 the body. Similarly, **myoglobin**, another iron-containing protein, helps deliver oxygen to muscle cells. Even if someone isn't anaemic, low ferritin levels (a marker of iron stores) can cause unexplained **fatigue**. Adequate iron intake may help manage fatigue. Iron plays a role in **muscle function** and energy metabolism. It's necessary for athletes and active individuals to maintain optimal iron levels for peak performance.

Electrolytes: Hydration and Beyond

Sodium, Potassium, and Chloride

Sodium: The salty sentinel—critical for nerve transmission and fluid balance. Sodium helps regulate fluid balance in the body. It ensures that the right amount of water stays inside and outside our cells. Proper fluid balance is essential for blood pressure regulation, nerve function, and overall cellular health. Sodium is vital for transmitting nerve signals and muscle contractions. Without sufficient sodium, our nerves wouldn't fire properly, leading to impaired movement and coordination. Sodium works alongside other electrolytes (such as potassium) to maintain blood pressure. It helps control blood volume 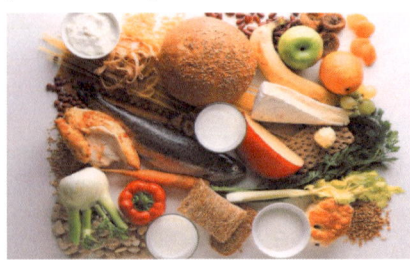 by affecting the amount of water in our blood vessels. When sodium levels are too high, the kidneys excrete more sodium, reducing blood volume. Conversely, when sodium levels are too low, the kidneys retain sodium to increase blood volume. Healthy kidneys play a significant role in maintaining consistent sodium levels. They adjust the amount of sodium excreted in urine to keep the body in balance. When sodium consumption and loss are not in equilibrium, it affects the total sodium concentration in the blood.

Potassium: The heart's ally—regulating heartbeat and muscle function. Potassium helps regulate fluid balance within our cells and throughout our bodies. This balance ensures proper hydration, nerve function, and overall cellular health. Remember, while potassium is 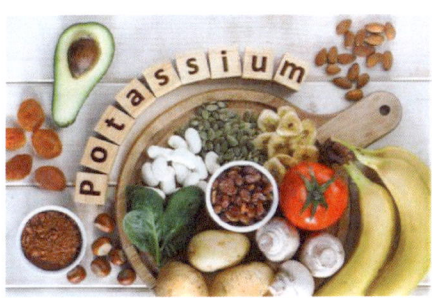 essential, excessive intake (often from processed foods and excessive salt) can lead to health issues. Striking the right balance is key—enough to support bodily functions but not too much to harm our health. So, enjoy potassium-rich foods like bananas, apricots, and potatoes, and let this often-neglected nutrient contribute to your well-being!

Chloride: The unsung hero of digestion and acid-base balance. Often overshadowed by its more famous counterpart, sodium, is a mineral that plays a vital role in maintaining our overall health. Chloride helps regulate fluid balance within our cells and throughout our bodies. It ensures that the right amount of water stays inside and outside our cells. Alongside sodium, chloride plays a crucial role in maintaining blood pressure. It affects blood volume by influencing water levels in our blood vessels. When chloride levels are too high, the kidneys excrete more chloride, reducing blood volume. Conversely, when chloride levels are too low, the kidneys retain chloride to increase blood volume. Chloride is crucial for the production and release of 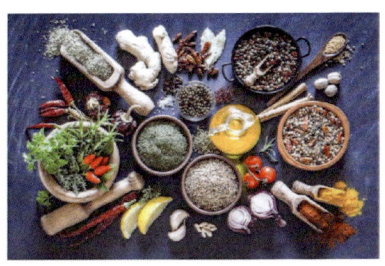 hydrochloric acid (HCl) in the stomach. Without HCl, foods couldn't be properly digested and absorbed. It also plays a role in maintaining the body's pH balance, ensuring that our internal environment remains stable. Chloride assists red blood cells in exchanging oxygen and carbon dioxide. It helps in both the lungs (taking up oxygen and releasing carbon dioxide) and other parts of the body (delivering oxygen and taking up carbon dioxide).

Mineral-Rich Foods: Nature's Multivitamins

From Spinach to Seaweed to Nuts and Seeds.

- **Spinach:** Popeye's secret weapon—packed with iron and magnesium. Spinach, a vibrant leafy green, is a nutritional powerhouse packed with essential nutrients. Here's why including spinach in your diet is a smart choice: Spinach is rich in vitamins and minerals, Vitamin A Spinach is high in carotenoids, which your body can convert into vitamin A. This vitamin supports eye health and immune function.

Vitamin C, A powerful antioxidant that promotes skin health and immune function. Vitamin K1 Essential for blood clotting; one spinach leaf contains over half of your daily needs. Folic Acid (Vitamin B9) Vital for normal cellular function and tissue growth. Iron Helps create haemoglobin, which transports oxygen to tissues. Calcium Essential for bone health and 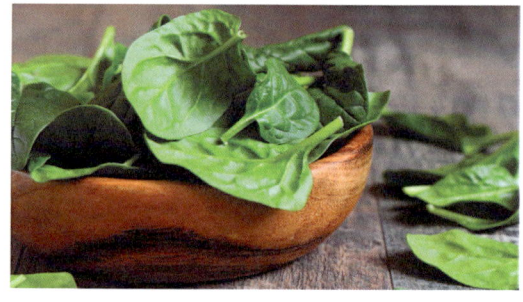 nervous systemfunction. Spinach is rich in plant compounds – Lutein Linked to improved eye health. Kaempferol An antioxidant that may decrease cancer risk. Nitrate Promotes heart health. Quercetin Fights infection and inflammation. Helps in Cancer prevention, Spinach's plant compounds may help ward off cancer. Helps with Bone health, Spinach's nutrients aid normal brain functioning.

- **Seaweed**: The ocean's treasure chest—abundant in iodine and trace minerals. Seaweed, also known as sea vegetables, offers a plethora of health benefits. It supports thyroid function, Seaweed contains iodine, a crucial mineral for proper thyroid function. Your thyroid gland relies on iodine to produce hormones that regulate growth, energy, and cell repair. Just one dried sheet of seaweed can provide 11-1,989% 0f the recommended daily iodine intake. It is rich in vitamins and minerals, A mere 1 tablespoon (7 grams) of dried spirulina can provide up to 20 calories, 4 grams of protein which is 11% of daily value in Iron, and 47% daily value in copper. It has many antioxidant properties and helps in gut health and weight management.

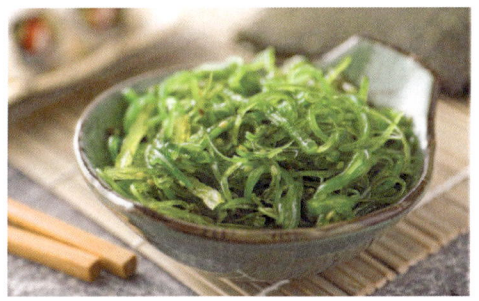

- **Nuts and Seeds:** Tiny powerhouses—delivering zinc, selenium, and more. Nuts and seeds are packed with essential nutrients. They provide plant protein, dietary fibre, and heart-healthy mono- and polyunsaturated fats. These little powerhouses also contain vitamins (such as vitamin E), minerals (like magnesium, phosphorus, copper, and manganese), and various plant compounds with antioxidant and anti-inflammatory properties. It takes care of your heart health, Regular consumption of nuts and seeds is associated with a lower risk of high blood pressure, cardiovascular disease (CVD), and even cancer. Clinical trials suggest that nuts may improve cholesterol and triglyceride levels, as well as reduce insulin resistance and oxidative stress. It helps you also prevent chronic diseases including diabetes. Their nutrient profile supports overall health and helps manage blood sugar levels.

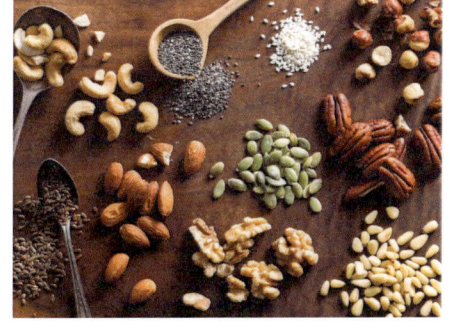

Athletes' Nutrient Demands

Fuelling the Fire Within

1. **Increased Needs**: Athletes sweat out minerals; they need replenishment.
2. **Supplements with Caution**: Whole foods first; supplements second.
3. **Timing Matters**: Pre-workout, post-workout—optimize mineral intake.

Minerals and Performance Enhancement

Beyond the Treadmill

1. **Zinc**: Boosting immunity and muscle repair.
2. **Copper**: Collagen synthesis for joint health.
3. **Manganese**: Enzymatic magic for energy production.

Minerals in Fitness isn't just about numbers on a label; it's about tapping into Earth's ancient wisdom. So, sip your coconut water, savor those leafy greens, and remember: **In these hidden gems, we find strength, resilience, and the essence of life itself.**

Phytonutrients: The Vibrant Guardians of Health

Nature's secret harmonies—found in colourful fruits and veggies.

Nature's Palette

From Carotenoids to Flavonoids

1. **Carotenoids**: Sun-kissed pigments—think carrots, tomatoes, and sweet potatoes. They're not just pretty; they protect our eyes, boost immunity, and dance with antioxidants.
2. **Flavonoids**: The orchestra of colours—found in berries, tea, and dark chocolate. They serenade our hearts, fight inflammation, and whisper tales of longevity.

Antioxidant Ballet

Free Radicals Beware

1. **Quenching Flames**: Phytonutrients wield antioxidant swords, neutralizing free radicals—the unruly troublemakers behind aging and disease.
2. **Resveratrol**: The grapes, berries and peanuts virtuoso—guarding our hearts and perhaps unlocking the secrets of longevity. The skins and seeds of grapes and berries contain resveratrol, which contributes to its particularly high concentration in red wine. Although much of the research has been done using supplements with high levels of resveratrol, it has shown promising health benefits. Here are some key points about resveratrol:

A: **Blood Pressure**: Resveratrol may help lower blood pressure by increasing the production of nitric oxide, which causes blood vessels to relax.

B: **Blood Fats**: Studies in animals suggest that resveratrol supplements may positively affect blood fats, including reducing total cholesterol levels and increasing "good" HDL cholesterol.

C: **Antioxidant Properties**: Resveratrol acts as an antioxidant, neutralizing free radicals and protecting against aging and disease.

Beyond the Salad Bowl

Let's get to know a bit more about Spices, Herbs, and Superfoods

- **Turmeric: We call it The Golden Healer**—Turmeric, the spice that gives curry its vibrant yellow colour, offers a multitude of health benefits.

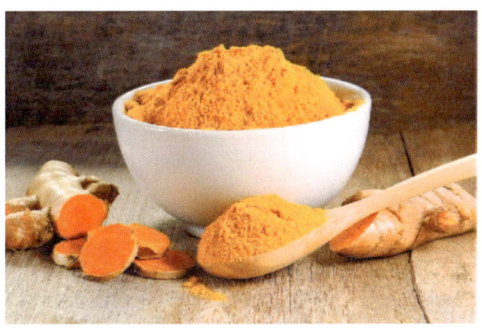

1. **Bioactive Compounds and Antioxidant Properties of Turmeric:**
   a) Turmeric contains curcuminoids, with curcumin being the most important.
   b) Curcumin is a potent antioxidant that neutralizes free radicals, protecting against oxidative damage.
   c) Although turmeric itself has only around 1-6% curcumin, supplements with higher curcumin content are more effective.
   d) To enhance curcumin absorption, consume it with black pepper (which contains piperine) or alongside a high-fat meal.

2. **Natural Anti-Inflammatory Effects:**
   a) Curcumin fights inflammation, making it potentially valuable in preventing and treating various health conditions.
   b) Chronic inflammation plays a role in many diseases, and curcumin's anti-inflammatory properties are beneficial.

3. **Boosts Antioxidant Capacity:**
   a) Turmeric helps combat oxidative stress, which contributes to aging and various diseases.
   b) By neutralizing free radicals, curcumin supports overall health.

4. **Heart Health and Cognitive Function:**
   a) Turmeric may reduce the risk of heart disease and improve cognitive function.
   b) Its anti-inflammatory and antioxidant effects play a role in these benefits.

5. **Potential Cancer Protection:**
   a) Curcumin shows promise in protecting against certain cancers.

    b) Research is ongoing, but its anti-inflammatory properties may inhibit cancer cell growth.

6. **Type 2 Diabetes Support**:
    a) Curcumin may help manage blood sugar levels and reduce insulin resistance.
    b) It contributes to overall metabolic health.

7. **Other Benefits**:
    a) Turmeric supports liver function, provides pain relief, and aids digestion.
    b) Its phytochemicals fight inflammation and oxidative stress, while vitamin C boosts immunity

Remember to incorporate turmeric into your diet creatively—whether in curries, teas, or golden milk—to reap its remarkable health benefits!

- **Garlic: Known as The pungent knight**—sword-fighting cholesterol and vampires alike. Garlic, that aromatic bulb with a pungent kick, offers an array of health benefits. Let's explore these:

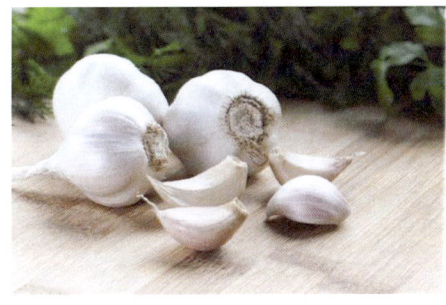

1. **Medicinal Properties**:
    - Garlic belongs to the Allium family (alongside onions, shallots, and leeks).
    - When you chop, crush, or chew garlic, it forms sulphur compounds like allicin.
    - Allicin is a potent antioxidant with various health benefits.
    - Other compounds, such as diallyl disulfide and s-allyl cysteine, also contribute to its effects.

2. **Nutrient-Rich and Low-Calorie**:
   - Calorie for calorie, garlic is a nutritional powerhouse.
   - A single clove (about 3 grams) contains:
     - Calories: 4.5
     - Protein: 0.2 grams
     - Carbs: 1 gram
     - Plus, it's rich in vitamin C, vitamin B6, and manganese.

3. **Immune System Boost**:
   - Aged garlic extract (AGE) can enhance your immune system.
   - Research suggests that AGE supplements reduce the severity of cold and flu symptoms.

4. **Heart Health**:
   - Garlic has long been associated with heart benefits.
   - Chemicals like **allicin** may help lower blood pressure and cholesterol levels.

5. **Other Notable Benefits**:
   - Eases common cold symptoms.
   - Supports bone health.
   - Removes heavy metal toxins.
   - Optimizes gut microflora.
   - May reduce dementia risk.
   - Enhances athletic performance.

Remember, garlic isn't just for warding off vampires—it's a flavourful ally for your well-being!

- **Green Tea: The zen master**—brewing tranquillity and catechins. Green tea, one of the healthiest beverages on the planet, offers a range of potential health benefits:

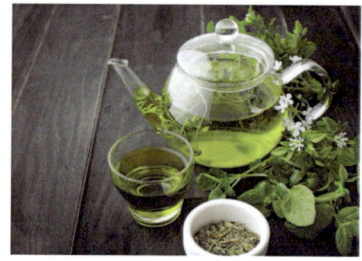

1. **Antioxidant Powerhouse**:
   - Green tea contains polyphenol antioxidants, including the well-known catechin called epigallocatechin-3-gallate (EGCG).
   - These antioxidants help prevent cell damage and offer various health benefits.

2. **Cognitive Function Enhancement**:
   - Compounds in green tea, such as caffeine and L-theanine, may benefit cognition, mood, and brain function.
   - Some studies suggest a lower chance of cognitive impairment in middle-aged and older adults who consume green tea.

3. **Fat Burning Potential**:
   - Green tea may increase metabolic rate and enhance fat burning, especially when paired with exercise.
   - While its overall effect on weight loss is likely small, it can still contribute to a healthier metabolism.

4. **Cancer Protection**:
   - Research links green tea consumption to a reduced risk of certain cancers, such as lung and ovarian cancer.
   - However, more high-quality human studies are needed to explore this further.

5. **Brain Aging Prevention**:
   - Green tea has been associated with lower levels of markers related to Alzheimer's disease in individuals without cognitive issues.
   - Compounds like EGCG and L-theanine may play a role in brain health.

Remember to enjoy your cup of green tea—it's not only refreshing but also beneficial for your well-being!

Phytoestrogens: This is your, Hormonal Harmony!

Soy, Flax, and Balance

1. **Soy Isoflavones**: The oestrogen mimics—finding equilibrium in menopause and beyond. **Isoflavones**, also known as **phytoestrogens**, are plant-based compounds found predominantly in beans, particularly **soybeans**. These remarkable molecules mimic the action of the hormone **oestrogen** within our bodies. The main isoflavones in soy are **genistein** and **daidzein**. When we consume soy, our intestinal bacteria break it down into these active forms. Once inside our bodies, soy isoflavones dock onto the same receptors as oestrogen, influencing various cellular processes. Soy's unique blend of **weak estrogenic** and **anti-estrogenic** activity makes it a fascinating addition to our diets. So, the next time you savor that soy sauce, remember that you're not just enjoying a savoury flavour—you're also benefiting from its subtle hormonal dance.

2. **Flaxseeds**: Tiny omega-3 warriors—shielding hearts and soothing hot flashes. **Flaxseeds**, also known as **linseeds**, are tiny nutritional powerhouses that have been cherished for centuries. Flaxseeds are one of the world's oldest crops, available in both brown and golden varieties. They offer a wealth of nutrients, Help in Protein which is Essential for tissue repair and overall health. Provides you with Fibre, Omega-3 fatty acids, and Thiamine (Vitamin B1)

The Art of Culinary Alchemy

Cooking with Magic

1. **Rainbow Plating**: Arrange your plate like a canvas—spinach, peppers, and blueberries.
2. **Herb Symphony**: Basil, oregano, thyme—season with love and phytonutrient flair.

In these plant pigments, we find resilience, joy, and the very essence of life.

Your Gut Health is your Inner Garden,

Where Microbes Dance

Within us lies a bustling ecosystem—the gut microbiome. These tiny dancers influence our digestion, immunity, and even mood. Learn how to tend to this garden, sowing probiotics, and prebiotics for a flourishing inner world.

Intuitive Eating: Listening to Hunger and Satiety

The Wisdom Within

Diets fade, intuition endures. Intuitive eating invites us to listen—to our growling stomachs, our cravings, our joy in savouring a ripe peach. It's not about restriction; it's about connection—with food and our own cues.

Plant-Based Nutrition: Green Alchemy

From Soil to Soul

Plants offer magic—a kaleidoscope of colours, flavours, and nutrients. We'll explore leafy greens, and the alchemy of turning plants into nourishment.

Spoiler alert: Plants are superheroes in disguise.

Sustainable Choices: Feeding Earth and Self

Beyond Our Plates

Nourishment extends beyond our bodies. It embraces the Earth—the soil, the oceans, the bees. Seasonal produce, reducing food waste, and honouring the interconnectedness of all life.

Conclusion

Nutrition Nourishment isn't a rigid rulebook; it's a love letter to food, health, and joy. So, let's raise our forks, sip our herbal teas, and honour the miracle of nourishment. Remember: **You're not just eating; you're weaving your own symphony of wellness.**

Chapter 4

Has Ashwagandha gained significant attention in Bodybuilding?

Ashwagandha, an adaptogenic herb from Ayurveda, also known as "Indian Winter Cherry" has indeed gained significant attention in scientific research, and has gained popularity for its potential benefits in **bodybuilding**. People have used ashwagandha for thousands of years to relieve stress and increase energy levels. Let's explore how it can positively impact bodybuilders:

1. **Stress Reduction and Anxiety Relief**:
   - Ashwagandha is renowned for its stress-relieving properties. Numerous studies have highlighted its ability to reduce stress and anxiety levels significantly.
   - Additionally, it has been linked to improved sleep quality, which contributes to better overall well-being.

2. **Blood Sugar and Fat Management**:
   - Small clinical trials have found that ashwagandha can help lower blood glucose levels and reduce triglycerides (common blood fats).
   - In fact, its blood sugar-lowering effects have been compared to those of medications prescribed for type 2 diabetes.

3. **Testosterone Boost and Muscle Growth**:
   - Ashwagandha plays a crucial role in **testosterone production**. For instance:

Has Ashwagandha gained significant attention in Bodybuilding?

- In infertile men, a daily dose of 5g of ashwagandha root powder led to a 13-22% increase in testosterone after just 3 months of use.
- Another study showed that infertile men given 3g of ashwagandha root extract experienced a testosterone increase of 14-41%.

4. **Cognition and Athletic Performance**:
   ○ Ongoing research suggests that ashwagandha may positively impact cognitive function and athletic performance.

5. **Safety and Side Effects**:
   ○ Generally, ashwagandha is considered safe, with minor possible side effects. However, caution should be exercised when using it alongside certain drugs.

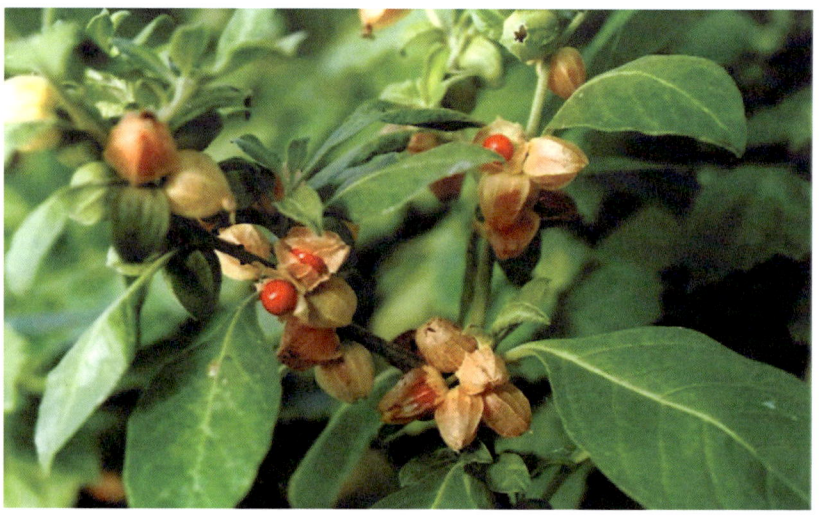

Herbal remedies have garnered interest due to their historical use and perceived natural origins. Educational intervention is an important factor, it bridges the gap between acceptance and knowledge.

We train to build our muscles and eat to feed those muscles, but do we ever stop to think about the health of our innards?

Ashwagandha may help bodybuilders by reducing stress, controlling cortisol, boosting testosterone, and supporting muscle growth. As with any supplement, consult a healthcare professional or dietician before incorporating it into your regime.

In summary, while herbal remedies continue to be used globally, their acceptance and scientific understanding remain areas of ongoing exploration.

Chapter 5

The Plateau and Perseverance

Breaking Through Plateaus: The Art of Perseverance in Fitness

Weeks turned into months. Progress slowed. The scale stalled. Doubt crept in. But my journal reminded me of victories past. I read about the day I ran my first mile without stopping, the morning I deadlifted my body weight, and the evening I turned down dessert. I pressed on, knowing plateaus were part of the journey.

In the exhilarating journey of fitness, plateaus emerge like stubborn roadblocks. These moments—when progress stalls and motivation wavers—test our resolve. But fear not! Welcome to *Breaking Through Plateaus: The Art of Perseverance in Fitness*, where we explore the science, mindset, and strategies to conquer these plateaus and reignite your fitness flame.

Understanding the Plateau

When Progress Hits Pause

What is a Fitness Plateau? It's that frustrating juncture when results seem elusive despite our best efforts.

The Three Reactions:

1. **Quit**: The siren call of defeat.
2. **Maintain**: Stagnation—the comfort zone.
3. **Adapt**: The path of perseverance.

Reasons Behind the Plateau

Intensity, Boredom, and Training Partners.

a) **Intensity Adjustment**: Our bodies adapt; it's time to shake things up. Modify workout intensity, introduce intervals, or tweak lifting tempo.

b) **Boredom and Repetitiveness**: The mind craves novelty. Change your routine, explore different classes, and reignite the spark.

c) **Training Partners**: Solo workouts can be demoralizing. Train with friends; let friendly competition propel you forward.

Mindset Matters

The Mental Gym

a) **Positive Spirit**: Believe nothing can derail your goals. Show up consistently, give your best, and allow proper recovery.

b) **Visualize Progress**: Imagine your future self—the stronger, fitter version. Let that vision fuel your perseverance.

Nutrition and Recovery

Fuel and Rest

a) **Nutrition**: Feed your body well. Balance macros, hydrate, and nourish with nutrient-dense foods.

b) **Rest and Sleep**: Recovery is part of progress. Prioritize quality sleep and allow muscles to repair.

Holistic Fitness

a) **Celebrate Small Wins**: Each rep, each session counts.

b) **Learn from Plateaus**: They reveal weaknesses. Address them.

c) **Community Support**: Train with others; witness progress together.

Perseverance turns roadblocks into stepping stones toward greatness.

Mind, Muscle, & Motion

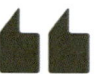

EAT BREAKFAST LIKE A LION,
LUNCH LIKE A TIGER,
EVENING MEAL LIKE A BEAR,
AND DINNER LIKE A WOLF.

SAHEEB DADAN

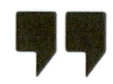

Chapter 6

The Myths of Fitness & Bodybuilding.

You ever come across Myths of bodybuilding and Fitness? I am sure we all hear this every day; Let's debunk some common Fitness & bodybuilding myths:

1. **Myth: It's Impossible to Stay Ripped Year-Round.**
   - **Fact**: Contrary to common belief, it is possible to stay ripped year-round. Maintaining a lean physique involves conscious eating and avoiding overeating. Your metabolism adapts as you lose weight, naturally decreasing hunger. So, even at low body fat percentages, you can stay lean and healthy.

2. **Myth: You Cannot Build Muscle and Burn Fat Simultaneously.**
   - **Fact**: While it's challenging, it's not impossible. Proper nutrition, resistance training, and adequate recovery allow for muscle gain while losing fat. Focus on a balanced approach and consistency.

3. **Myth: Clean Bulking Prevents Fat Gains.**
   - **Fact**: Clean bulking (gradual calorie surplus with nutrient-dense foods) doesn't guarantee zero fat gain. Excess calories, even from healthy sources, can lead to fat accumulation. Monitor your intake and adjust as needed.

The Myths of Fitness & Bodybuilding.

4. **Myth: Everyone Is on Steroids or PEDs.**
   - **Fact**: While some bodybuilders use performance-enhancing drugs (PEDs), not everyone does. Many achieve impressive results naturally through hard work, proper training, and nutrition.

5. **Myth: You Need Supplements.**
   - **Fact**: Supplements aren't mandatory. A well-balanced diet provides essential nutrients. While supplements can be helpful, they're not a substitute for real food.

6. **Myth: You Need to Eat Healthy to Get Lean.**
   - **Fact**: While healthy eating is beneficial, achieving leanness is primarily about managing caloric intake. You can get lean while enjoying occasional treats, as long as you stay within your calorie limits.

7. **Myth: You Need to Lift Heavy to Build Muscle.**
   - **Fact**: Both heavy and moderate weights can stimulate muscle growth. Focus on progressive overload, proper form, and consistency. Rep ranges matter less than overall effort.

8. **Myth: All Hollywood Actors Are Juicing.**
   - **Fact**: While some actors may use PEDs for movie roles, not all do. Genetics, hard work, and professional trainers contribute to their transformations.

9. **Myth: Carbs are bad for Weight Loss.**
   - **Fact**: Carbohydrates are essential for energy. Choose whole grains, fruits, and vegetables for sustained energy and overall health.

10. **Myth: More is Better.**
    - **Fact**: Overtraining can lead to injury and imbalances. Find a balanced plan that includes healthy eating, cardio, resistance training and mobility work.

11. **Myth: No Pain No Gain.**
    - **Fact**: While some discomfort during exercise is normal, extreme pain can indicate an injury. Listen to your body and avoid pushing through severe pain.

12. **Myth: Yoga is just stretching.**
    - **Fact**: Yoga combines strength, flexibility, balance, and mindfulness. It's more than just stretching – it's holistic practise for physical and mental well-being.

Chapter 7

How do the Myths in Fitness impact you as an Athlete?

Myths can indeed infiltrate the mind, affecting our mindset and approach to fitness. Let's explore how these myths can take hold:

1. **False Expectations**:
    - Myths create unrealistic expectations. When we believe in quick fixes or magical solutions, we set ourselves up for disappointment.
    - Unrealistic expectations can lead to frustration, self-doubt, and a negative mindset.

2. **Comparison Trap**:
    - Bodybuilding myths often involve comparing ourselves to others—whether it's their progress, physique, or methods.
    - Constant comparison can erode confidence and make us feel inadequate.

3. **Fear of Deviation**:
    - Myths create rigid rules. When we fear deviating from these rules, we limit our flexibility and adaptability.
    - Fear of straying from the myth can lead to anxiety and mental rigidity.

4. **Obsession with Perfection**:
    - Myths often promote an idealized version of fitness. We chase perfection, fearing any deviation.
    - This obsession can lead to anxiety, overtraining, and burnout.

5. **Self-Criticism**:
   - Believing myths can make us hypercritical of our progress. We focus on perceived flaws rather than celebrating achievements.
   - Self-criticism erodes self-esteem and motivation.
6. **All-or-Nothing Mindset**:
   - Myths often present extreme approaches (e.g., "no pain, no gain"). We adopt an all-or-nothing mindset.
   - This mindset can lead to guilt when we miss a workout or indulge in a treat.
7. **Loss of Joy**:
   - Myths can make fitness feel like a chore. We forget the joy of movement and focus solely on results.
   - Losing joy in the process affects our mental well-being.

Remember, critical thinking and evidence-based knowledge are essential. Challenge myths, seek accurate information, and prioritize a positive, balanced mindset in your fitness journey!

The iron temple awaits, where myths crumble and gains ascend.

Chapter 8

What is the secret behind a Summer body?

Picture this, you perched on a sun-kissed beach, your six pack abs glistening like a freshly polished trophy. As you sip your coconut water, beachgoers gather in awe. Children point, their ice cream cones forgotten. Elderly couples nudge each other, whispering, "Remember when we had abs like that?" Even the sand crabs pause their scuttling, their tiny claws forming a standing ovation.

The lifeguard usually stoic, blows his whistle and approaches you "Sir, he says, squinting at your chiselled midsection, I'm afraid your abs are violating the beach's 'No Excessive Hotness Policy."

You chuckle, flexing a bicep. "I apologize. It's genetic." Haha

A nearby women's volleyball game grinds to a halt. The ball hands mid-air, suspended by sheer admiration. Suddenly, all these women start walking towards you, just then the coconut water slips out of your hand and spills on to your abs, and your eyes open and your dream comes to an end.

So! Was the summer body a mere dream? Fear not my friend, summer bodies are sculpted in all seasons.

The concept of a **"summer body"** has been perpetuated by media, diet culture, and fitness marketing. Let's delve into the secrets and implications behind it:

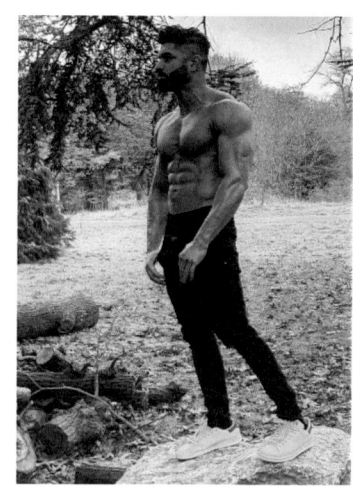

1. **What Is a Summer Body?**
    - A **"summer body"** is often portrayed as an idealized

beauty standard: a flat stomach, toned physique, devoid of cellulite or stretch marks. It's the image perpetuated by diet culture and fitness industries year-round.
- Specifically, during summer, there's pressure to achieve this **homogenous** and **Eurocentric** figure. The term implies that warmer weather necessitates peak physical form, emphasizing body fat loss and toning.

2. **The Impact of the Term:**
   - The phrase **fuels toxic beauty ideals** and encourages thinness. It implies that to enjoy summer or be seen as attractive, bodies must conform to a specific appearance.
   - Weight stigma associated with the concept can lead to disordered eating, sleep disturbances, and alcohol use.
   - Healing our relationship with our bodies and food involves seeking professional help and finding supportive communities.

3. **The Reality:**
   - Achieving a **"summer body"** is not a one-size-fits-all goal. Bodies come in diverse shapes and sizes, and true health encompasses mental, emotional, and physical well-being.
   - Instead of chasing an elusive ideal, focus on **self-care, movement**, and **nourishing** your body year-round.
   - Remember that everybody is a **summer body** when it enjoys the warmth, sunshine, and experiences life fully, regardless of appearance.

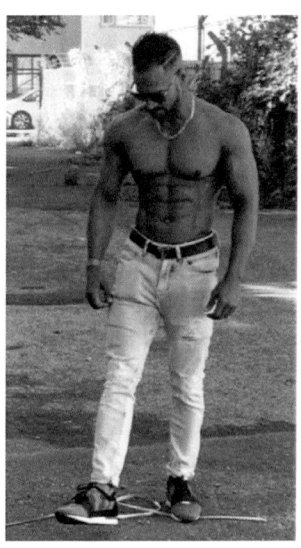

In essence, prioritize self-love, acceptance, and holistic health over external standards. Your body deserves care and appreciation, no matter the season!

What is the secret behind a Summer body?

How do you achieve this summer body?

Achieving a **summer body** involves a combination of **healthy habits** and **consistent effort**. Here are some steps to help you get started:

1. **Stay Hydrated:**
    - Proper hydration is essential. Drinking enough water boosts your metabolism, reduces hunger, and supports overall health. Consider using an **infuser water bottle** to make hydration more interesting by adding fruits like strawberries, berries, oranges, lemons, or limes.
    - As an Athlete you should drink at least minimum 3 litres of water a day.

2. **Summer Body Diet:**
    - Focus on **real food** that nourishes your body. Eat less processed and packaged foods.
    - Learn to cook quick, healthy, and nutritionally balanced meals.
    - Prioritize fresh fruits, vegetables, lean proteins, whole grains, and healthy fats.

3. **Summer Body Workout:**
    - Regular exercise is crucial. Aim for a mix of **cardiovascular** and **strength training** exercises.
    - Incorporate activities like running, swimming, cycling, or dancing.
    - Strength training helps build muscle and boost metabolism. Include bodyweight exercises, dumbbell workouts, or resistance training.

4. **Get Enough Sleep:**
    - Quality sleep is essential for recovery, muscle growth, and overall well-being.
    - Aim for 7-9 hours of restful sleep each night.

5. **Eat Enough Protein:**
   - Protein supports muscle repair and growth. Include sources like chicken, fish, tofu, beans, and Greek yogurt.

6. **Reduce Stress Levels:**
   - Chronic stress can impact weight and overall health. Practice relaxation techniques such as meditation, yoga, or deep breathing.

7. **Record Your Progress:**
   - Keep track of your journey. Take photos, note your workouts, and celebrate small victories.

Remember, a **summer body** is not about achieving a specific look but feeling confident, healthy, and energized. Embrace the process and enjoy the journey!

Chapter 9

How do Cheat Meals impact your fitness journey?

Cheat meals play an interesting role in the world of bodybuilding. Let's explore how they impact your fitness journey:

1. **Strategic Importance:**
   - **Cheat meals** are a tantalizing break from strict dietary routines. Even renowned bodybuilders like Dwayne "The Rock" Johnson indulge in burgers, pizza, or pasta laden with fat and cheese while maintaining their enviable physiques.
   - Esteemed trainers like George Farah and Dave Palumbo incorporate cheat meals into bodybuilding programs strategically.

2. **How Cheat Meals Work:**
   - Our bodies adapt to certain calories and nutrients over time. A regular clean diet can lead to stagnation.
   - **Cheat meals** disrupt this adaptation by introducing sudden high-calorie portions with fat, carbs, and protein that our bodies aren't used to.
   - Replenishing glycogen stores during cheat meals provides energy for the following week, and surprisingly, the body responds better.

3. **Types of People and Cheat Meals:**
   - **Obese (Fat Loss):** For non-bodybuilders, a cheat meal with high calories (e.g., a burger and fries or pizza) can be beneficial without excessive protein.

- **Getting in Shape (Fit or Physique):** Include more protein in your cheat meal (e.g., pizza with chicken BBQ). Feeding your muscles along with high calories is essential.
- **Bodybuilders (Offseason):** Opt for high-density meals or days. If you're already on high-calorie days, consider an open buffet or a protein-rich cheat meal.

Cheat meals can be a useful tool when used correctly. They reset hormones, replenish glycogen, and keep calorie-burning mechanisms active. So, enjoy that occasional indulgence!

What are the benefits and the drawbacks of Cheat Meals?

Cheat meals can have both benefits and drawbacks for athletes, including strength athletes. Let's explore:

1. **Benefits of Cheat Meals:**
   - **Metabolic Reset:** Cheat meals can offset hormonal changes associated with hard dieting, helping to prevent a slowdown in metabolism.
   - **Psychological Relief:** Maintaining a strict diet requires significant willpower. A short break from the regimen can provide mental relief and rejuvenate motivation.
   - **Glycogen Replenishment:** Cheat meals replenish glycogen stores, providing increased energy for workouts.
   - **Positive Hormonal Impact:** When used correctly, cheat meals can reset hormones responsible for metabolism and insulin regulation.
2. **Drawbacks for Strength Athletes:**
   - **Performance Impact:** For strength athletes, maintaining optimal performance in the gym is crucial. If cheat meals negatively affect your training, they might not be the best choice.

How do Cheat Meals impact your fitness journey?

- **Balancing Act:** Your diet should be structured to ensure you feel your best during workouts. Frequent cheat meals could hinder performance.
- **Individual Considerations:** Assess how cheat meals affect your strength gains, recovery, and overall well-being. Some athletes may benefit more than others.

In summary, while cheat meals can be useful tools, it's essential to strike a balance. Listen to your body, monitor performance, and adjust accordingly. Remember, there's no one-size-fits-all approach!

Chapter 10
Is Beast mode all about Ego?

Beast mode—those two words echo like war drums, Summoning the warrior spirit, where weakness succumbs. It's not a switch you flip; it's a transformation complete, From mortal to titan, from defeat to victory's seat. In the gym's sacred temple, the iron bows down, as you lift, push, and grind—each rep a battle crown. Your veins surge with lightning, your sinews ignite, you're not merely lifting weights; you're claiming your right.

Beast mode isn't about ego; it's about discipline, The grind when no one's watching, the hunger deep within. It's the early morning sprints, the midnight protein shake, the sacrifice of comfort for the gains you'll make.

When doubt knocks on your door, tell it to wait outside, for you're in beast mode, and there's no place to hide. The weights become your allies, the mirror your witness, as you sculpt your destiny, relentless and fearless.

Beast mode is a multifaceted concept that extends beyond mere ego. Let's explore its dimensions:

1. **Physical Intensity:**
    - Beast mode often refers to pushing your physical limits during workouts or challenges. It's about giving your all, regardless of external factors.
    - While ego might play a role in wanting to prove yourself, the true essence lies in dedication, discipline, and relentless effort.

2. **Mindset and Focus:**
   - Beast mode transcends ego when you channel your mental energy toward a goal. It's about unwavering focus, mental resilience, and determination.
   - Ego-driven actions might seek validation, but beast mode seeks self-improvement and growth.

3. **Discipline and Consistency:**
   - Beast mode demands consistency, whether it's hitting the gym, practicing a skill, or pursuing excellence.
   - Ego-driven actions can be sporadic, seeking short-term gains. Beast mode thrives on long-term commitment.

4. **Humility and Learning:**
   - True beast mode involves humility. It's acknowledging that there's always more to learn, more to achieve.
   - Ego often resists learning, assuming it already knows everything.

5. **Support and Community:**
   - Beast mode isn't a solitary pursuit. It thrives within a supportive community—training partners, coaches, or mentors.
   - Ego isolates and The beast mode connects.

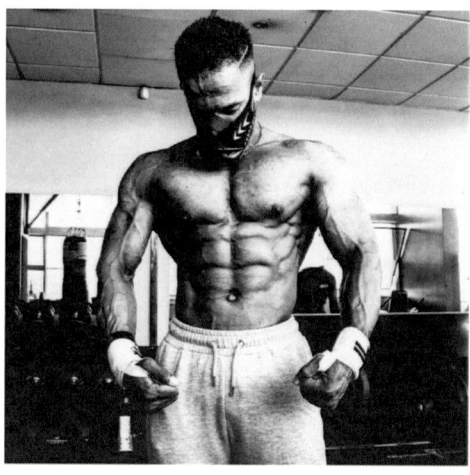

Roar like a lion, let the echoes pierce the sky, forge your body, your mind, and let mediocrity die. In the crucible of effort, you'll find your true form, A beast unchained, a force of nature, a thunderstorm.

Remember, it's not about perfection; it's about the fight, The hunger that burns brighter when the day turns to night. Embrace the struggle, wear your scars like a badge, for in beast mode, you're writing an epic, not a footnote on a page.

So go forth, dear reader, with fire in your eyes, In the arena of life, where the mighty beast lies. Unleash your power, defy the ordinary's code, for you're not just lifting weights—you're embodying **beast mode**.

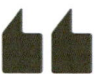

HEALTHY FOOD IS LIKE YOUR BANK ACCOUNT, THE MORE HEALTHY FOOD YOU EAT, THE MORE YOU INVEST IN YOUR HEALTH.

SAHEEB DADAN

Chapter 11

Training Routine for Beginners, Intermediaries and Advanced.

Workout for beginners:

As a beginner, it's essential to start with exercises that build a solid foundation and help you develop proper form. Here are some basic training workouts I started with, perhaps you can try:

1. **Bodyweight Squats**:
   - Stand with your feet shoulder-width apart.
   - Lower your body by bending your knees and hips, as if sitting back into an imaginary chair.
   - Keep your chest up and your back straight.
   - Return to the starting position by pushing through your heels.
   - Aim for 20 repetitions.

2. **Push-Ups**:
   - Start in a plank position with your hands slightly wider than shoulder-width apart.
   - Lower your body by bending your elbows, keeping them close to your sides.
   - Push back up to the starting position.
   - Modify by doing knee push-ups if needed.
   - Aim for 10 repetitions.

Training Routine for Beginners, Intermediaries and Advanced.

3. **Walking Lunges**:
    - Take a step forward with your right leg, lowering your body until both knees are bent at 90 degrees.
    - Push off your right foot to return to the standing position.
    - Repeat with your left leg.
    - Aim for 10 lunges per leg.

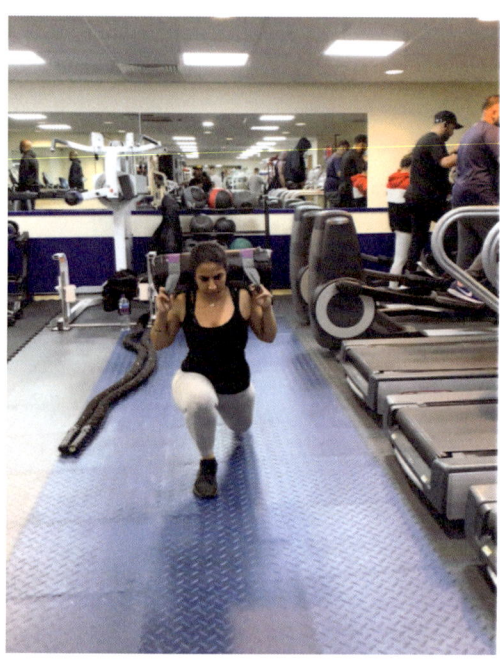

4. **Dumbbell Rows** (using a light dumbbell):
    - Stand with your feet hip-width apart, holding a weight in your right hand.
    - Bend forward at the hips, keeping your back straight.
    - Pull the weight toward your hip, squeezing your shoulder blades together.
    - Lower the weight back down.
    - Aim for 10 repetitions per arm.

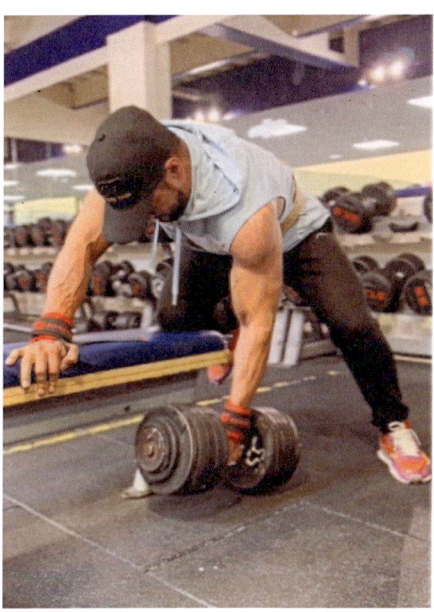

5. **Planks**:
    - Start in a push-up position, but with your weight on your forearms.
    - Keep your body in a straight line from head to heels.
    - Hold this position for 15 seconds.
    - Gradually increase the duration as you get stronger.

6. **Jumping Jacks**:
    - Stand with your feet together and arms by your sides.
    - Jump, spreading your legs wide and raising your arms overhead.
    - Jump again to return to the starting position.
    - Aim for 30 jumping jacks.

7. **Treadmill**:
    - Walk for the first 10 minutes.
    - Start increasing your speed gradually for the next 20 minutes.
    - Put the treadmill machine on incline between 6-12.
    - Last 10 minutes finish it by walking on a normal speed.

Training Routine for Beginners, Intermediaries and Advanced.

Remember to warm up before your workout and cool down afterward. As you progress, gradually increase the intensity, and add more exercises to your routine. Listen to your body, stay consistent, and enjoy your fitness journey! 💪

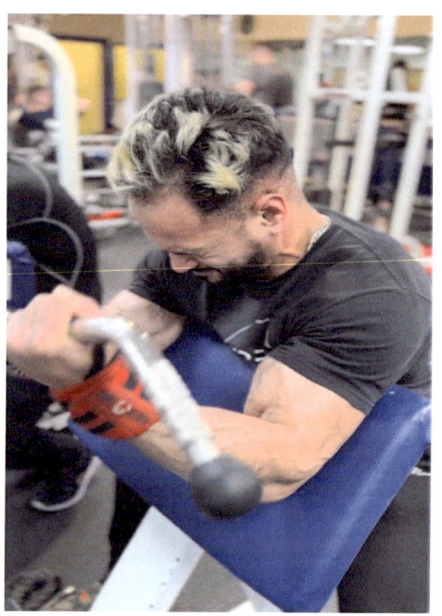
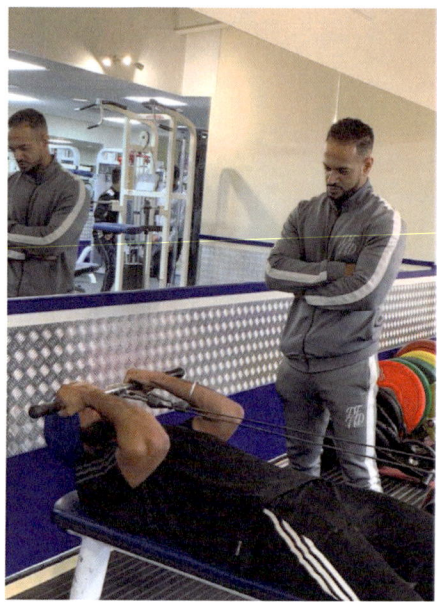

Workout for Intermediaries:

As an intermediate lifter, you're ready to take your fitness journey to the next level. Here's an **8-week workout program** designed specifically for intermediates. Remember to maintain proper form and gradually increase weights as you progress:

Monday Workout: Upper Body

1. **Incline Barbell Bench Press**:
    - Warm-up: 2 sets of 12 reps
    - Working sets: 3 sets of 8-12 reps
2. **Dumbbell Bench Press**:
    - 3 sets of 8-12 reps

3. **Wide Grip Pullup**:
   - Warm-up: 2 sets of 12 (use pull-down machine if needed)
   - Working sets: 3 sets to failure
4. **Bent-Over Barbell Row**:
   - 3 sets of 8-12 reps
5. **Seated Dumbbell Press**:
   - Warm-up: 1 set of 12 reps
   - Working sets: 3 sets of 8-12 reps
6. **Dumbbell Side Lateral Raise**:
   - 3 sets of 8-12 reps
7. **Sit-Ups**:
   - 3 sets of 20 reps

Tuesday Workout: Lower Body
1. **Barbell Curl**:
   - Warm-up: 1 set of 12 reps
   - Working sets: 3 sets of 8-12 reps
2. **Lying Triceps Extension**:
   - 3 sets of 8-12 reps
3. **Standing Calf Raise**:
   - 3 sets of 8-12 reps
4. **Barbell Back Squat**:
   - Warm-up: 2 sets of 12 reps
   - Working sets: 3 sets of 8-12 reps
5. **Dumbbell Lunge**:
   - 3 sets of 8-12 reps
6. **Barbell Romanian Deadlift**:
   - Warm-up: 1 set of 12 reps
   - Working sets: 3 sets of 8-12 reps

Training Routine for Beginners, Intermediaries and Advanced.

7. **Hanging Leg Raise**:
   - 3 sets of 20 reps

Wednesday Off Day
Thursday Workout: Upper Body (Different Focus)

1. **Barbell Bench Press**:
   - Warm-up: 2 sets of 12 reps
   - Working sets: 3 sets of 8-12 reps

2. **Incline Dumbbell Bench Press**:
   - 3 sets of 8-12 reps

3. **Close Grip Pull-Up**:
   - Warm-up: 2 sets of 12 (use pull-down machine)
   - Working sets: 3 sets to failure

4. **Cable Row**:
   - 3 sets of 8-12 reps

5. **Barbell Upright Row**:
   - Warm-up: 1 set of 12 reps
   - Working sets: 3 sets of 8-12 reps

6. **Military Press**:
   - 3 sets of 8-12 reps

7. **Floor Crunch**:
   - 3 sets of 20 reps

Friday Workout: Lower Body (Different Focus)

1. **Seated Dumbbell Curl**:
   - Warm-up: 1 set of 12 reps
   - Working sets: 3 sets of 8-12 reps

2. **Weighted Dip**:
   - 3 sets of 8-12 reps

3. **Seated Calf Raise**:
    - 3 sets of 8-12 reps
4. **Barbell Front Squat**:
    - Warm-up: 2 sets of 12 reps
    - Working sets: 3 sets of 8-12 reps
5. **Leg Press**:
    - 3 sets of 8-12 reps
6. **Lying Leg Curl**:
    - 1 set of 12 reps
    - Working sets: 3 sets of 8-12 reps
7. **Lying Leg Raise**:
    - 3 sets of 20 reps

Remember to rest adequately between sets and stay consistent. Adjust weights as needed and enjoy your fitness journey! 💪🏋️

Workout for Advanced Lifters:

As an advanced lifter, you're ready to take your fitness to the next level. Here are two effective workout programs designed for advanced lifters:

1. **The Ultimate 8-Week Workout for Advanced Lifters**:
    - This program focuses on increasing frequency, volume, and intensity. Perform the following workout twice per week:
    - **Day 1 (Upper Body)**:
        - Incline Bench Press: 4 sets of 8-12 reps
        - Dumbbell Bench Press: 4 sets of 8-12 reps
        - Dumbbell Fly: 3 sets of 10-12 reps
        - Wide Grip Pullup: 4 sets to failure (use pull-down machine if needed)
        - Bent-over Barbell Row: 4 sets of 8-12 reps
        - Narrow Grip Pull Down: 3 sets of 10-15 reps

Training Routine for Beginners, Intermediaries and Advanced.

- Hanging Leg Raise: 3 sets of 20 reps
- Crunch: 3 sets of 20 reps

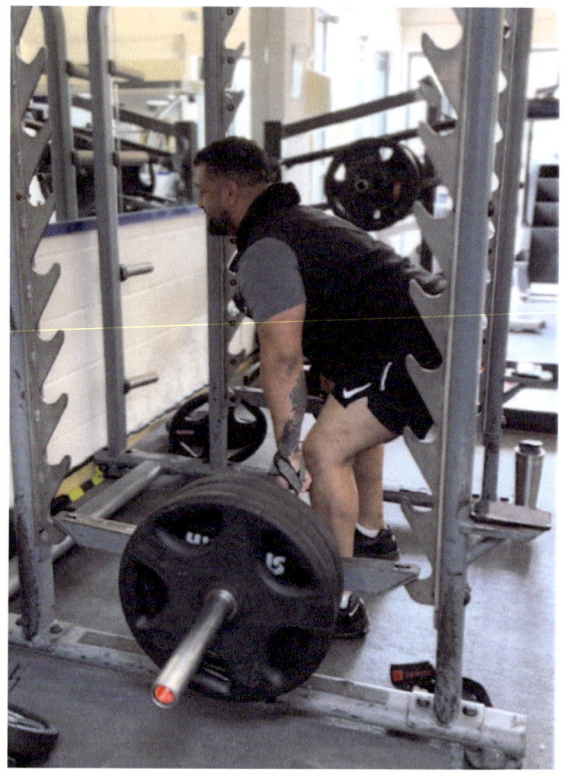

- **Day 2 (Upper Body)**:
  - Seated Dumbbell Press: 4 sets of 8-12 reps
  - Dumbbell Lateral Raise: 3 sets of 10-15 reps
  - Bent Over Rear Lateral Raise: 3 sets of 10-15 reps
  - Barbell Curl: 4 sets of 8-12 reps
  - Weighted Dip: 4 sets of 8-12 reps
  - Seated Dumbbell Curl: 4 sets of 8-12 reps
  - Incline Dumbbell Curls: 4 sets of 8-12 reps
  - Decline Sit Up: 3 sets of 20 reps
  - Lying Leg Raise: 3 sets of 20 reps

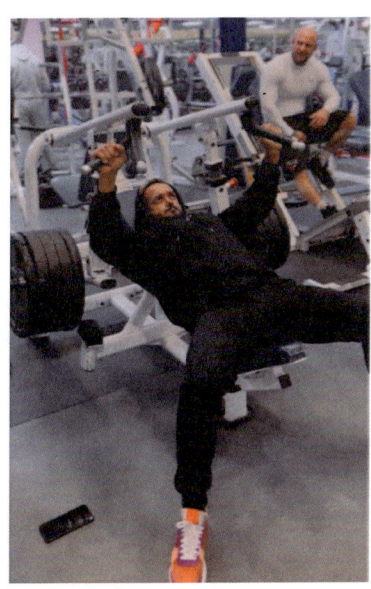

- ○ **Day 3 (Lower Body)**:
  - ➤ Standing Calf Raise: 3 sets of 10-15 reps
  - ➤ Seated Calf Raise: 3 sets of 10-12 reps
  - ➤ Leg Press: 4 sets of 10-15 reps
  - ➤ Barbell Back Squat: 3 sets of 8-12 reps
  - ➤ Dumbbell Walking Lunge: 3 sets of 10-15 reps
  - ➤ Barbell Romanian Deadlift: 3 sets of 8-12 reps
  - ➤ Lying Leg Curl: 3 sets of 8-12 reps

2. **(a) Advanced Bodybuilder Workout**:
   - ○ This program targets each muscle group once a week over 5 days:
     - ➤ Monday: Shoulders
     - ➤ Tuesday: Arms
     - ➤ Wednesday: Legs
     - ➤ Thursday: Back
     - ➤ Friday: Chest
     - ➤ Plus, add 1 abdominal exercise at the end of each daily workout.

Training Routine for Beginners, Intermediaries and Advanced.

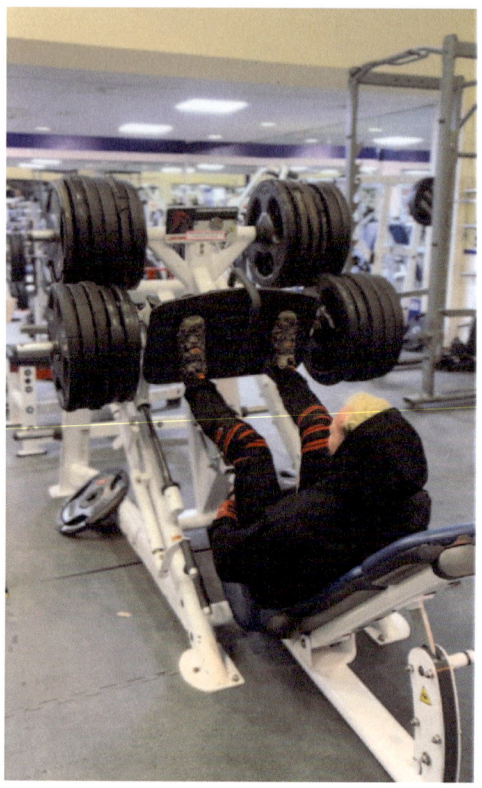

(b) Advanced Bodybuilder Workout:
- This program targets each muscle group over 6 days:
  - Monday: Quads
  - Tuesday: Chest
  - Wednesday: Back, Abs & Calves
  - Thursday: Shoulders, Traps & Hamstrings
  - Friday: Biceps, Triceps, Abs & Calves
  - Saturday: Back

Remember to adjust weights, rest adequately between sets, and stay consistent. Enjoy your challenging workouts and keep pushing your limits! 💪🏋

Chapter 12
My Ultimate Abs Workout routine.

Ultimate Abs Workout:

Strengthening your core is essential for overall fitness and functional movement. Building strong and defined abs requires a combination of targeted exercises and consistency. It takes time, dedication, and hard work to get those packs. The exercises below have helped me stand out on stage and bring out the best 6 packs on me. These are some of the **best ab exercises** to target different areas of your midsection and help you achieve that chiselled core:

1. **Barbell Floor Wiper**:
   - Lie on your back with your arms extended, holding a barbell above your chest.
   - Lift your legs off the ground and move them side to side, like a windshield wiper.
   - Engages obliques and lower abs.

2. **Medicine Ball Slam**:
   - Stand with knees slightly bent, holding a medicine ball overhead.
   - Slam the ball down to the ground with force.
   - Works your entire core and builds explosive power.

3. **Side Jackknife**:
   - Lie on your side, legs extended.
   - Lift your legs and upper body simultaneously, reaching for your toes.
   - Targets obliques and improves stability.

My Ultimate Abs Workout routine.

4. **Hanging Knee Raise**:
   - Hang from a pull-up bar.
   - Bend your knees and lift them toward your chest.
   - Excellent for lower abs.

5. **Machine Crunch**:
   - Use a cable machine with a rope attachment.
   - Kneel and pull the rope down toward your thighs, crunching your abs.
   - Adds resistance for a stronger core.

6. **Pallof Press**:
   - Stand sideways to a cable machine.
   - Hold the handle at chest level and extend your arms.
   - Resist the cable's pull by engaging your core.
   - Enhances stability and anti-rotation strength.

7. **Planks**:
   - Get into a push-up position, but with your weight on your forearms.
   - Keep your body in a straight line from head to heels.
   - Hold this position for as long as you can (aim for at least 30 seconds).

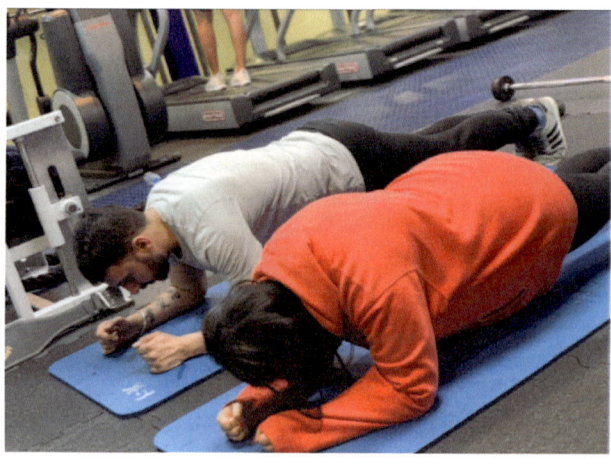

8. **Russian Twists**:
    - Sit on the floor with your knees bent and feet lifted.
    - Hold a weight or medicine ball.
    - Twist your torso to the right, then to the left, tapping the weight on the ground each time.

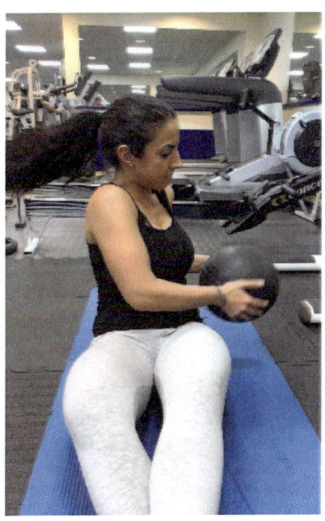

9. **Leg Raises:**
    - Lie on your back with your hands under your hips.
    - Lift your legs off the ground, keeping them straight.
    - Lower them back down without touching the floor.

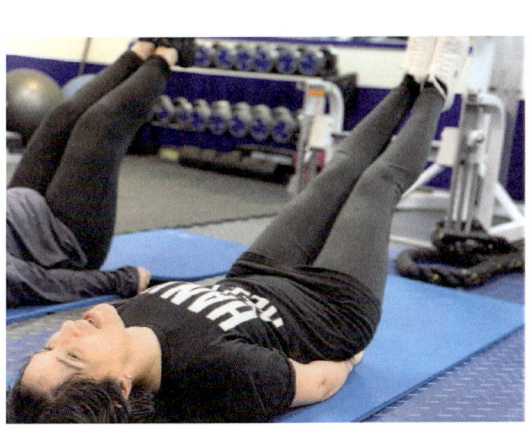
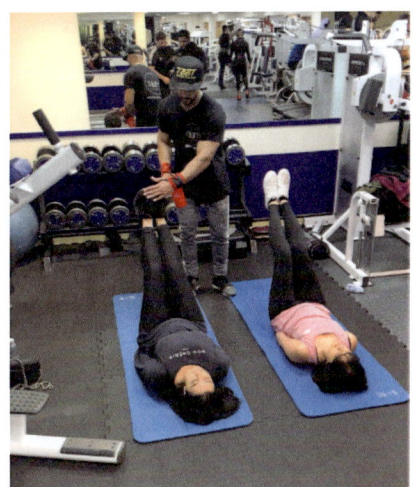

My Ultimate Abs Workout routine.

10. **Bicycle Crunches:**
    - Lie on your back with your hands behind your head.
    - Bring your right elbow to your left knee while extending your right leg.
    - Alternate sides in a cycling motion.

11. **Hanging Leg Raises:**
    - Hang from a pull-up bar.
    - Lift your legs straight up toward your chest.
    - Lower them back down slowly.

12. **Mountain Climbers:**
    - Start in a push-up position.
    - Alternate bringing your knees toward your chest in a running motion.

13. **Ab Wheel Rollouts:**
    - Kneel on the floor with an ab wheel or stability ball in front of you.
    - Roll forward, extending your arms, and then roll back up.

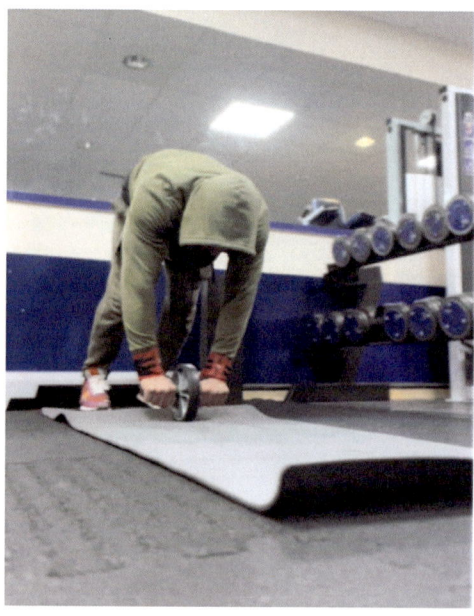

Mind, Muscle, & Motion

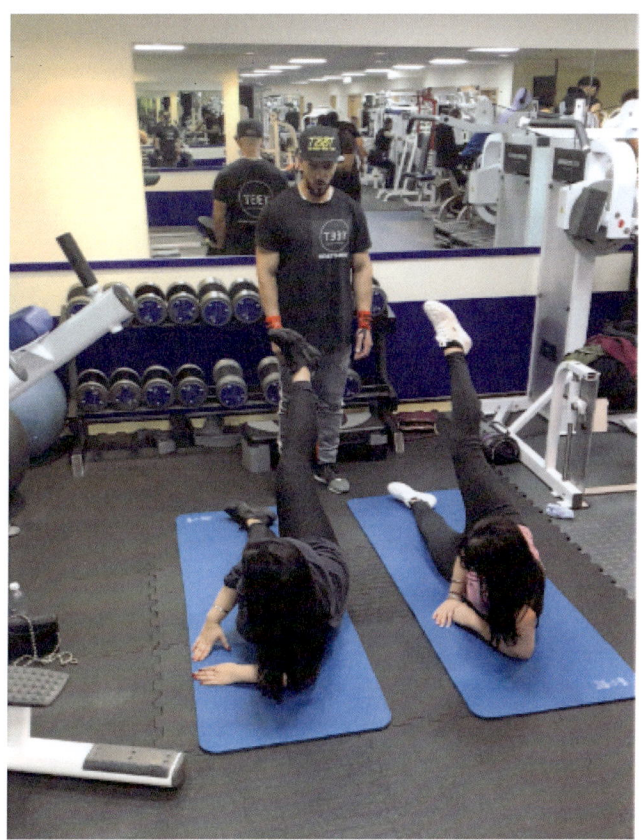

    Remember to mix and match these exercises to create a well-rounded ab workout. Consistency and proper form are key! Focus on quality over quantity. Perform these exercises with proper form and gradually increase the intensity. Combine them with a healthy diet and overall fitness routine for the best results! 💪

Chapter 13

Are supplements more important than food in bodybuilding?

A **well-balanced diet** should provide most of the nutrients you need for bodybuilding, **supplements** can be a useful addition to support your nutrition plan. However, it's important to remember that supplements should **not replace a healthy diet** and should be used in consultation with a healthcare professional or a registered dietitian.

Let's explore this further:

1. **Food is always first**:
   - **Food** is the foundation of any nutrition plan. It provides essential macronutrients (carbohydrates, proteins, and fats) and micronutrients (vitamins and minerals).
   - Whole foods offer a wide range of nutrients, fibre, and phytochemicals that contribute to overall health and well-being.

2. **Supplements as Complements**:
   - **Complementary Role**: Supplements can fill gaps in your diet when certain nutrients are lacking or when specific goals (such as muscle building) require additional support.
   - **Convenience**: Supplements offer convenience, especially for busy individuals who may struggle to meet their nutritional needs solely through food.

3. **Common Supplements in Bodybuilding**:
   - **Protein**: While whole foods are excellent sources of protein, protein supplements (such as whey or casein) can be convenient for post-workout recovery and muscle growth.

It helps in weight loss as well as muscle building. For Weight Loss, consuming protein can increase the number of calories burned (boosting your metabolic rate) and reduce appetite, aiding in weight loss. If you want to gain or maintain muscle, most studies suggest 1.0 – 2.2 grams of protein per kilogram of body weight.

- **Creatine**: Creatine monohydrate is well-researched and can enhance strength and performance during resistance training. Creatine is an energy booster for muscles. Supports your muscle growth and boosts the formation of proteins that increase muscle fibre size and raises levels of insulin-like growth factor (IGF-1). Also improves your high intensity exercise performance and speeds up your muscle growth.

- **BCAAs (Branched-Chain Amino Acids)**: These amino acids (leucine, isoleucine, and valine) play a role in muscle protein synthesis. Specifically, the BCAA leucine activates a pathway that stimulates muscle protein synthesis, aiding in muscle development. BCAAs decreases muscle growth and prevents muscle wasting, BCAAs are crucial for preserving muscle mass.

- **Multivitamins**: A good multivitamin can help cover any micronutrient gaps in your diet. It not only helps your immune system support but also helps in filling nutritional gaps. They help fill gaps caused by limited diets or impaired nutrient absorption.

- **Omega-3 Fatty Acids**: Fish oil supplements provide essential fatty acids important for overall health. Promotes brain health during pregnancy and early life. Omega-3s reduce the risk of heart attacks and strokes. Include omega-3-rich foods like fatty fish (salmon, mackerel, sardines), flaxseeds, chia seeds, and walnuts in your diet.

4. **Considerations**:
   ○ **Individual Needs**: Everyone's nutritional requirements are different. Factors like age, gender, activity level, and health conditions influence nutrient needs.
   ○ **Quality Matters**: Not all supplements are created equal. Choose reputable brands and consult professionals for guidance.
   ○ **Safety**: Some supplements may interact with medications or have side effects. Always consult a healthcare provider.

In summary, prioritize whole foods, but use supplements strategically to enhance your bodybuilding journey. Remember that no supplement can replace a well-rounded diet and consistent training!

Chapter 14

The basics of diet plan.

Every individual's body is unique, and factors such as genetics, metabolism, lifestyle, and health conditions play a significant role in how our bodies respond to diet and exercise. Here are some reasons why personalized diet plans are essential:

1. **Metabolism:**
    - People have varying metabolic rates. Some burn calories quickly, while others have a slower metabolism.
    - A personalized diet considers your metabolic needs and adjusts calorie intake accordingly.

2. **Body Composition:**
    - Different people have varying proportions of muscle, fat, and water.
    - A diet plan should align with your body composition goals (e.g., fat loss, muscle gain).

3. **Activity Level:**
    - Sedentary individuals require fewer calories than active ones.
    - Your daily activity level influences your energy needs.

4. **Health Conditions:**
    - Conditions like diabetes, hypertension, or food allergies impact dietary choices.
    - Personalized plans accommodate specific health needs.

5. **Food Preferences and Tolerances:**
    - Some people love certain foods, while others dislike them.

The basics of diet plan.

- A good diet plan considers your preferences and avoids foods you can't tolerate.

6. **Nutrient Requirements:**
   - Age, gender, and life stage (e.g., pregnancy, breastfeeding) affect nutrient needs.
   - Personalized plans ensure adequate vitamins, minerals, and macronutrients.

7. **Goals:**
   - Weight loss, muscle gain, athletic performance—everyone has different objectives.
   - Customized plans align with your specific goals.

8. **Behavioural Patterns:**
   - Some people thrive on structured meal plans, while others prefer intuitive eating.
   - Personalization considers your behavioural tendencies.

9. **Psychological Factors:**
   - Emotional eating, stress, and social influences impact dietary choices.
   - A personalized plan addresses these factors.

10. **Long-Term Sustainability:**
    - A diet you can stick to is more effective than short-term fads.
    - Personalized plans promote sustainable habits.

In summary, **one-size-fits-all** diets rarely work. Consulting a registered dietitian or nutritionist can help create a personalized plan that suits your body, preferences, and lifestyle.

Remember that health is a journey, and individualization is key!

Basic Weekly Weight Loss Programme.

Are you struggling to lose weight? Spoke to a lot of trainers and friends and still no results? Let's get to the most basic diet plans. They say if nothing works get back to the basic.

If you're aiming to **lose weight**, it's essential to focus on a balanced diet that provides adequate nutrients while creating a calorie deficit. Here's a simple **7-day weight loss meal plan** to get you started:

Day 1: Balanced Start

- **Breakfast**:
    - Greek yogurt with berries and a sprinkle of almonds.
    - Whole-grain toast with avocado.
- **Lunch**:
    - Grilled chicken salad with mixed greens, cherry tomatoes, cucumber, and balsamic vinaigrette.
- **Dinner**:
    - Baked salmon with quinoa and steamed broccoli.

Day 2: Protein-Packed

- **Breakfast**:
    - Scrambled eggs with spinach and feta cheese.
    - Whole-grain toast.
- **Lunch**:
    - Lentil soup with a side of whole-grain bread.
- **Dinner**:
    - Turkey meatballs with zucchini noodles and marinara sauce.

Day 3: Plant-Based

- **Breakfast**:
    - Overnight oats with almond milk, chia seeds, and sliced banana.

- **Lunch**:
  - Chickpea salad with diced bell peppers, red onion, and lemon-tahini dressing.
- **Dinner**:
  - Roasted sweet potatoes stuffed with black beans, corn, and avocado.

Day 4: Mediterranean Flavors

- **Breakfast**:
  - Whole-grain toast with hummus and sliced cucumber.
- **Lunch**:
  - Greek salad with olives, feta cheese, and grilled chicken.
- **Dinner**:
  - Grilled shrimp with quinoa tabbouleh.

Day 5: Light and Fresh

- **Breakfast**:
  - Smoothie with spinach, banana, almond milk, and protein powder.
- **Lunch**:
  - Caprese salad (tomato, mozzarella, basil) drizzled with olive oil.
- **Dinner**:
  - Baked white fish with asparagus and lemon.

Day 6: High-Fiber Choices

- **Breakfast**:
  - Oatmeal topped with sliced strawberries and a dollop of peanut butter.

- **Lunch**:
  - Brown rice bowl with black beans, roasted veggies, and salsa.
- **Dinner**:
  - Grilled tofu with quinoa and stir-fried broccoli.

Day 7: Balanced Finish

- **Breakfast**:
  - Cottage cheese with pineapple chunks.
- **Lunch**:
  - Turkey and avocado wrap in a whole-wheat tortilla.
- **Dinner**:
  - Baked chicken breast with roasted Brussels sprouts.

Vegan Diet Plans.

Diet 1: Vegan

- **Breakfast**:
  - Dry Quinoa 60 grams with chia see 1 tsp and 70 grams mixed fruits.
- **Lunch**:
  - 250 grams of mushrooms with 80 grams red lentils.
- **Dinner**:
  - 500 gram Cauliflower with 70 gram brown rice and ground flax seed 2 tsp.
- **Snacks**:
  - Baby spinach 80 grams with nuts and raisin mix 1 ounce and 1 raw medium peach.

The basics of diet plan.

Diet 2: Vegan
- **Breakfast**:
  - 2-3 small oranges.
- **Lunch**:
  - Firm Tofu 170 gram with 1 tsp soya sauce and mixed salad of 150 gram.
- **Dinner**:
  - Sweet potatoes raw unprepared 400 gram with mushrooms 250 gram.
- **Snacks**:
  - Mixed nuts and raisins 1 ounce with 1 banana.

Diet 3: Vegan
- **Breakfast**:
  - 2-3 small oranges or raw plum.
- **Lunch**:
  - Tomato salad 150 gram with 2 carrots and 1 banana.
- **Dinner**:
  - Sweet potatoes raw unprepared 400 gram with Flax seed 2 tsp.
- **Snacks**:
  - Mixed nuts and raisins 1 ounce with raw parsnip 250 gram.

Diet 4: Vegan
- **Breakfast:**
  - 2-3 small oranges or raw plum.
- **Lunch**:
  - Tomato salad 150 gram with 2 carrots and 1 banana.

- **Dinner**:
  - 80 grams of Lobia salad with mix vegetables.
- **Snacks**:
  - Mixed nuts and raisins 1 ounce with raw parsnip 250 gram.

Remember to **stay hydrated**, control portion sizes, and include plenty of fruits, vegetables, lean proteins, and whole grains. Also, consider seeking professional advice.

Above is the most basic programme which has helped a lot of my clients in the past.

Basic Weekly Bulking Programme for Muscle gain.

If you're aiming to **bulk up** and gain lean muscle mass, a well-structured diet is crucial. Here's a **clean bulking diet plan** to help you maximize muscle growth while minimizing fat gain:

Understanding Bulking for Muscle Gain

- **What Is Bulking?**
  - Bulking refers to a phase of training where you intentionally increase your calorie intake to build muscle mass.
  - There are two types of bulks:
    - **Clean Bulks**: Prioritize healthy foods and aim to minimize fat gain while adding muscle.
    - **Dirty Bulks**: Involve eating anything to gain muscle, often leading to fat gain.

Key Aspects of Bulking

1. **Caloric Surplus**:
   - To build muscle, you must eat more calories than your body uses.
   - Calculate your maintenance level using a TDEE calculator and eat around 300-500 calories above that.

The basics of diet plan.

2. **Protein Intake**:
   - Protein is essential for muscle repair and growth.
   - Aim for adequate protein (about 1.2-2.2 grams per kilogram of body weight).
3. **Healthy Carbohydrates and Fats**:
   - Include complex carbs (whole grains, sweet potatoes) and healthy fats (avocado, nuts).
   - These provide energy for workouts and overall health.
4. **Strength Training**:
   - Lift heavy weights to stimulate muscle growth.
   - Progressive overload (increasing weight or reps) is essential.
5. **Cardio and HIIT**:
   - Incorporate moderate cardio to maintain cardiovascular health and aid fat loss.
   - High-Intensity Interval Training (HIIT) can be effective for fat burning.

Sample Clean Bulking Diet Plan

1. **Breakfast**:
   - Scrambled eggs with spinach and whole-grain toast.
   - Greek yogurt with berries.
2. **Mid-Morning Snack**:
   - Cottage cheese with almonds.
3. **Lunch**:
   - Grilled chicken breast with quinoa and steamed broccoli.
4. **Afternoon Snack**:
   - Protein shakes with almond milk and a banana.

5. **Dinner**:
    - Baked salmon with sweet potatoes and asparagus.
6. **Evening Snack**:
    - Greek yogurt with a drizzle of honey.

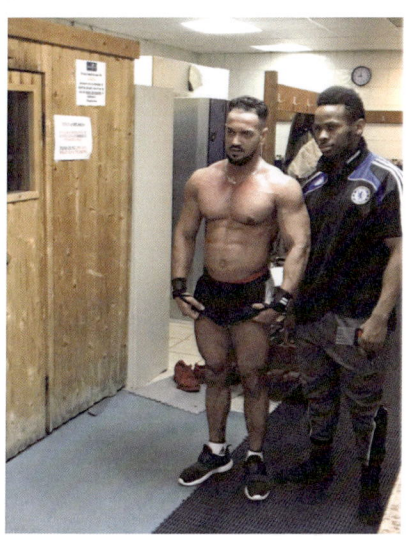

Hydration and Rest

- **Stay hydrated**: Water is essential for muscle function and recovery.
- **Get enough rest**: Muscles grow during rest, so prioritize sleep.

Remember, consistency and patience are key. Adjust portion sizes based on your individual needs and monitor progress. Consult a registered dietitian or nutritionist for personalized guidance. Happy bulking!

Chapter 15
The Get-Ripped Foods

As an Athlete, sticking to a diet and achieving that ripped physique means you need to be consuming certain foods every day, but that does not mean depriving your tastebuds. For more fun in your diet, try and swap these foods in your diet.

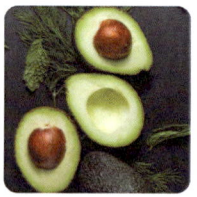

Fruit	Calories	Protein(g)	Carbs(g)	Fat(g)
Avocado 1/4	77	1	3	8

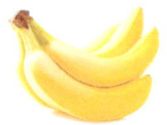

Fruit	Calories	Protein(g)	Carbs(g)	Fat(g)
Banana	53	1	14	tr

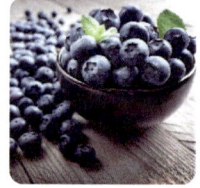

Fruit	Calories	Protein(g)	Carbs(g)	Fat(g)
Blueberries 1/2 cup	42	1	21	tr

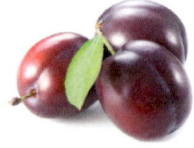

Fruit	Calories	Protein(g)	Carbs(g)	Fat(g)
Plums, 2 small	60	2	16	tr

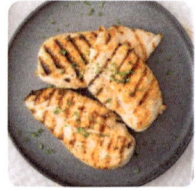

Meat/Fish/Poultry	Calories	Protein(g)	Carbs(g)	Fat(g)
Chicken Breast, 8 oz	250	50	0	5

Mind, Muscle, & Motion

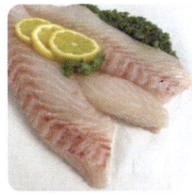

Meat/Fish/Poultry	Calories	Protein(g)	Carbs(g)	Fat(g)
Cod, 10 oz	233	51	0	2

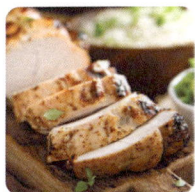

Meat/Fish/Poultry	Calories	Protein(g)	Carbs(g)	Fat(g)
Skindless Turkey, 3.5 oz	135	30	0	1

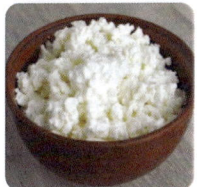

Milk/Egg	Calories	Protein(g)	Carbs(g)	Fat(g)
Cottage Cheese 1/2 Cup	80	14	3	1

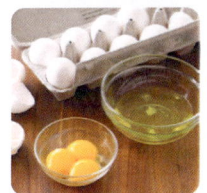

Milk/Egg	Calories	Protein(g)	Carbs(g)	Fat(g)
Egg White	17	4	tr	tr

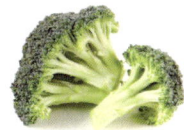

Vegetables	Calories	Protein(g)	Carbs(g)	Fat(g)
Broccoli	31	3	6	tr

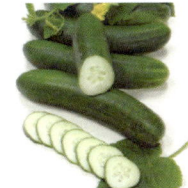

Vegetables	Calories	Protein(g)	Carbs(g)	Fat(g)
Cucumber, 1 cup chop	14	1	3	tr

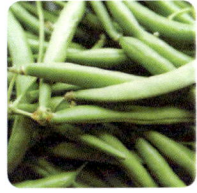

Vegetables	Calories	Protein(g)	Carbs(g)	Fat(g)
Green beans, 1 cup	34	2	8	tr

The Get-Ripped Foods

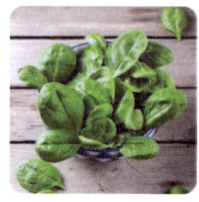

Vegetables	Calories	Protein(g)	Carbs(g)	Fat(g)
Spinach, 1/2 cup	7	1	1	tr

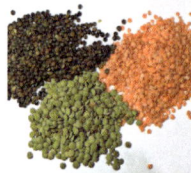

Legumes	Calories	Protein(g)	Carbs(g)	Fat(g)
Lentils. 1/2 cup cooked	115	9	20	tr

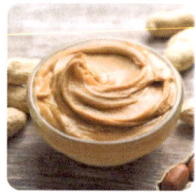

Nuts/Seeds	Calories	Protein(g)	Carbs(g)	Fat(g)
Peanut Butter 2 tbsp	190	8	6	tr

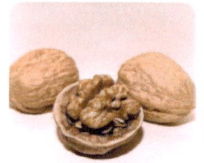

Nuts/Seeds	Calories	Protein(g)	Carbs(g)	Fat(g)
Walnuts	172	7	3	tr

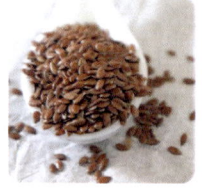

Nuts/Seeds	Calories	Protein(g)	Carbs(g)	Fat(g)
Flaxseeds	166	7	6	tr

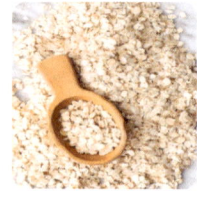

Nuts/Seeds	Calories	Protein(g)	Carbs(g)	Fat(g)
Oatmeal, 1 cup	150	6	25	2

When aiming to **get ripped** (achieve a lean and muscular physique), your diet plays a crucial role. Remember that getting ripped involves a combination of **nutrition**, **exercise**, and **consistency**. Pair your diet with an effective workout plan to achieve your desired results!

I LOAD MY LEG PRESS MACHINE FULL OF WEIGHTS, I SMILE, AND I PRESS THE HELL OUT OF IT.

SAHEEB DADAN

Chapter 16

The 8 golden rules to stay Ripped the whole year.

The Protein Powerhouse:
- Protein is your best friend on the path to ripped glory.
- It helps maintain and build lean muscle mass while keeping you full and satisfied.
- Opt for sources like chicken, turkey, fish, eggs, Greek yogurt, and tofu.

Quality Carbs:
- Don't fear carbs—they're essential for energy and recovery.
- Choose complex carbs like sweet potatoes, quinoa, brown rice, and oats.
- These keep your metabolism humming and prevent muscle breakdown.

Healthy Fats:
- Good fats are your allies. They enhance satiety and support overall health.
- Include avocados, nuts, seeds, and olive oil in your diet.
- They also help absorb fat-soluble vitamins like A, D, E, and K.

Hydration Heroes:
- Water isn't just for thirst—it's your secret weapon.
- Proper hydration aids digestion, boosts metabolism, and keeps your skin looking sharp.
- Guzzle that H_2O like it's the elixir of gains.

Micronutrients Matter:
- Vitamins and minerals are like tiny superheroes.
- They optimize cellular function, support recovery, and keep your immune system robust.
- Load up on colourful fruits, veggies, and leafy greens.

Timing Is Everything:
- Get a Pre-workout, grab a balanced meal with protein and carbs to fuel your session.
- Grab a post workout, refuel within an hour with protein and fast-digesting carbs to kickstart recovery.
- Nighttime Casein protein (from cottage cheese or Greek yogurt) helps repair muscles during sleep.

Portion Control:
- Even the healthiest foods can sabotage your goals if you overeat.
- Track your portions and stay within your calorie target.
- Remember, abs are made in the kitchen, not the all-you-can-eat buffet.

Consistency Wins:
- Getting ripped isn't a sprint; it's a marathon.
- Consistently choose nutrient-dense foods, stay active, and be patient.
- Rome wasn't shredded in a day, my friend.

So, load up on protein, embrace those veggies, and hydrate like a boss. Your ripped physique awaits!

The 8 golden rules to stay Ripped the whole year.

As some of us struggle to make our preps, here is an introduction for all of you readers to Fit Eat UK – Your Personalized Meal Prep Solution

Are you tired of spending hours in the kitchen, juggling work, family, and a healthy lifestyle? Look no further! At Fit Eat UK, we're passionate about making your life easier and healthier. Our mission is simple: to provide delicious, nutritious, and convenient meals that fit seamlessly into your busy schedule.

Why Choose Fit Eat UK?

1. **Tailored to Your Needs**: Whether you're a fitness enthusiast, a busy professional, or a health-conscious parent, these guys have got you covered. Their diverse menu caters to various dietary preferences, including Lean Bulk, Weight Loss, keto, gluten-free, and more.

2. **Quality Ingredients**: They believe that great meals start with great ingredients. That's why they source fresh, locally grown produce and high-quality proteins. No shortcuts, no compromises.

3. **Chef-Crafted Delights**: Their talented chefs blend culinary expertise with nutritional science to create mouthwatering dishes. From savoury breakfasts to hearty dinners, every bite is a celebration of flavour.

4. **Convenience Redefined**: Say goodbye to meal planning, grocery shopping, and cooking. With Fit Eat UK, your meals arrive at your doorstep – ready to heat and enjoy. It's like having a personal chef without the hefty price tag.

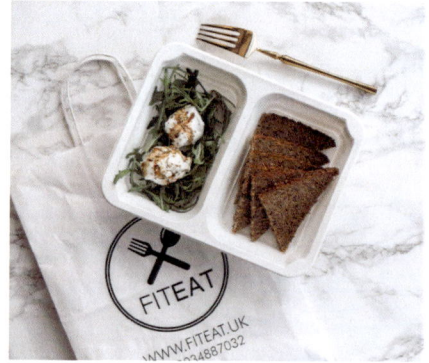

5. **Flexible Subscriptions**: Choose from weekly, bi-weekly, or monthly subscriptions. Adjust your menu, skip a week, or try new dishes – it's all about what works best for you. Fit Eat UK offers the following lengths of subscription: 3 days, 1 week, 2 weeks, 4 weeks, or 8 weeks. For 5 or 6 days a week. Also, you can order a trial day with them.

How It Works

1. **Browse & Order**: Explore their menu online. Select your favourite meals, snacks, and sides.
2. **Delivery**: They deliver your freshly prepared meals right to your home or office. No fuss, no hassle.
3. **Heat & Eat**: Pop your meal in the microwave or oven, and voilà! A gourmet experience in minutes.

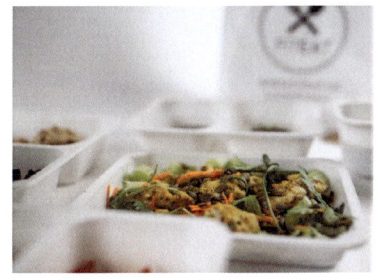

Below is a small Introduction from the Head Chef Tomasz Nowak and why Fit Eat UK is one of the best in the fitness Industry.

When was Fit Eat UK formed?

Fit Eat was founded in 2017, pioneering specialized meal plans offered on a subscription basis in London.

What does Fit Eat UK specialise in?

Fit Eat specializes in crafting diet meal plans tailored to meet the specific needs of individuals, ranging from 1300 kcal to up to 4000 kcal per day. Right now, we have 14 different diets in our offer to choose from.

The 8 golden rules to stay Ripped the whole year.

What made you start this journey of making prepped meals?

The inspiration behind launching Fit Eat stemmed from the absence of affordable meal providers offering comprehensive daily meal plans. Witnessing this gap, we embarked on the journey to establish a service that addressed this need. Today, we're gratified to have garnered a loyal customer base across London, with thousands of satisfied clients.

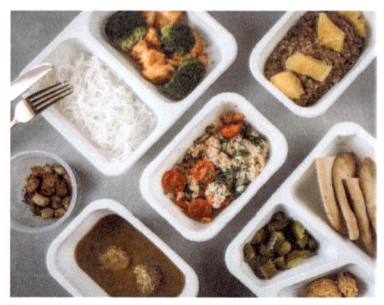

Do you customise the meals according to the needs of Athletes and Bodybuilders?

We do offer meal plans designed specifically for athletes and bodybuilders. Our High Protein and Bodybuilding VIP diet options prioritize the optimal balance of protein and carbohydrates in the diet. Depending on caloric requirements, we provide up to approximately 310g of protein per day.

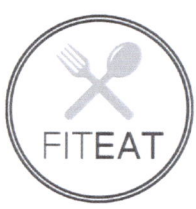

Do you deliver meals on a weekly basis?

Our meal delivery service operates on a daily basis.

Do you enjoy your job, as you are helping many Athletes and Bodybuilders?

Absolutely, we find immense joy in our work. Beyond fostering a friendly and familial environment within our company, we take pride in supporting our customers on their health journeys. This extends to athletes and bodybuilders, who constitute a significant portion of our clientele.

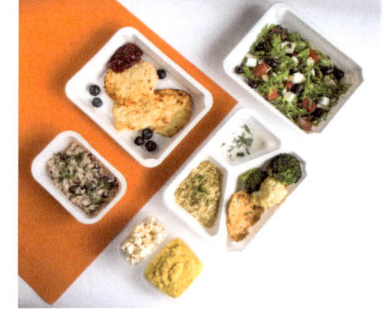

What advice do you have for all the readers when it comes to meals?

We believe in breaking the myth that eating healthy must be difficult and expensive. At Fit Eat UK, we're here to show that you don't need to spend hours in the kitchen or count every calorie. With our service, you can enjoy our tasty meals hassle-free, based on your preferences.

Join the Fit Eat UK Family.

Ready to reclaim your time and nourish your body? Join thousands of satisfied customers who've made Fit Eat UK their go-to meal prep solution. Let's make healthy eating effortless and enjoyable!

Visit their Instagram page fiteatuk to explore their menu and get started today. Contact: 020 3488 7032

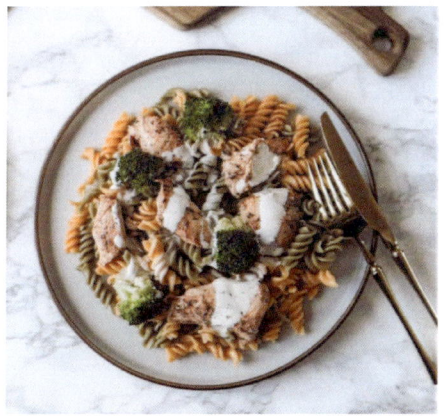

Chapter 17

Why is it so important to train with like-minded people?
(Community & Camaraderie)

I joined fitness classes and met like-minded souls. We sweated together, laughed together, and shared our struggles. My journal became a testament to these connections—the friendships forged over dumbbells and protein shakes. We cheered each other on, celebrating milestones big and small.

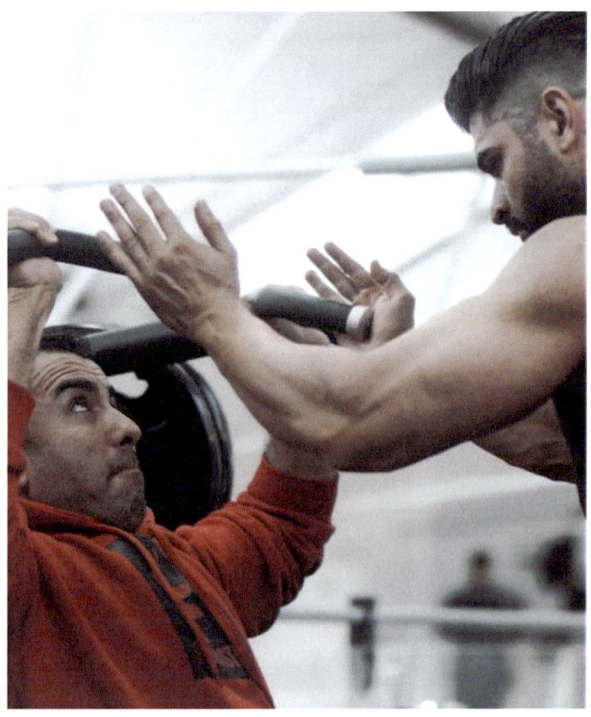

Training in the gym with like-minded people offers several benefits that can enhance your fitness journey. Let's explore why this camaraderie matters:

1. **Motivation and Accountability:**
   - Being surrounded by people who share your fitness goals provides motivation. You'll witness their dedication, which can inspire you to stay committed.
   - Accountability naturally arises when you train with others. You're less likely to skip workouts or give up when you know someone is expecting you.

2. **Shared Interests and Passion:**
   - Like-minded gym buddies share your passion for fitness. Conversations revolve around workouts, nutrition, and progress.
   - These shared interests create a positive environment where everyone supports each other.

3. **Friendly Competition:**
   - Healthy competition pushes you to perform better. When you see others working hard, you'll strive to match their effort.
   - Friendly challenges can elevate your workouts and lead to better results.

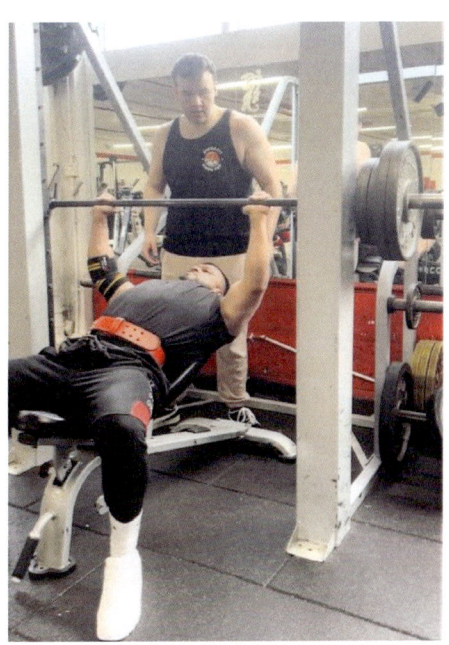

4. **Social Connection and Friendship:**
   - The gym becomes a social hub. You'll meet people who understand your lifestyle and appreciate your dedication.

(Community & Camaraderie)

- Building friendships with like-minded individuals fosters a sense of community and belonging.

5. **Knowledge Sharing:**
- Gym buddies exchange tips, techniques, and workout routines. You'll learn from their experiences and vice versa.
- This knowledge-sharing accelerates your progress and helps you avoid common pitfalls.

6. **Positive Energy and Fun:**
- Training with friends makes workouts enjoyable. Laughter, encouragement, and shared achievements create a positive atmosphere.
- Fun workouts are sustainable workouts!

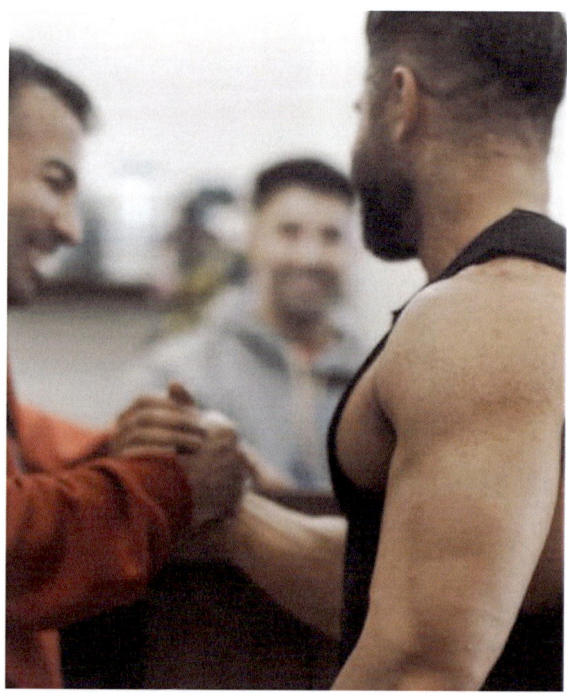

Remember, the gym isn't just about lifting weights—it's about building connections, supporting each other, and celebrating victories together!

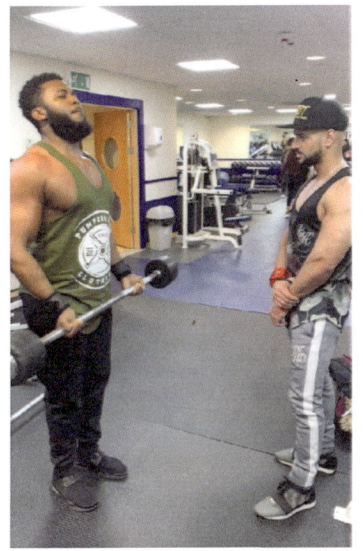 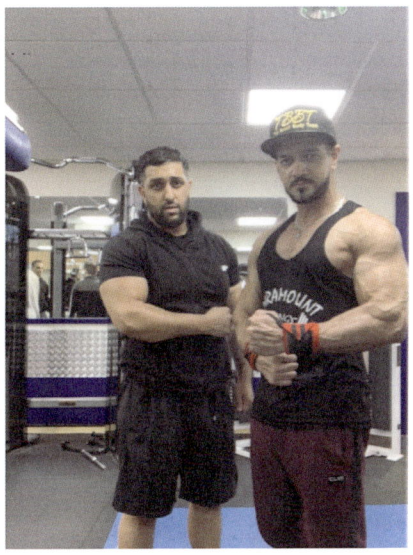

Training with No Weakness (Omar)   Bicep session with Umair

The Gym Spotters

    A spotter in the gym is like a trusty sidekick for weightlifters. They play a crucial role during weightlifting exercises by providing us assistance and ensuring safety. This is where your gym camaraderie comes in. I was always blessed to have such people around me. Friends are most useful when lifting heavy weights, think bench presses, squats, and deadlifts. When you are lifting like a power lifter, friends become your lifeline.

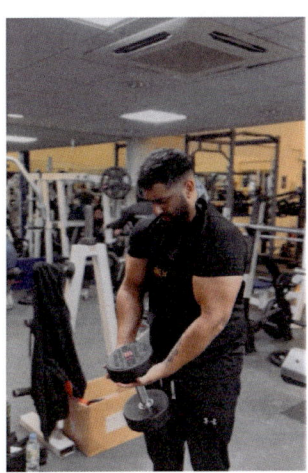 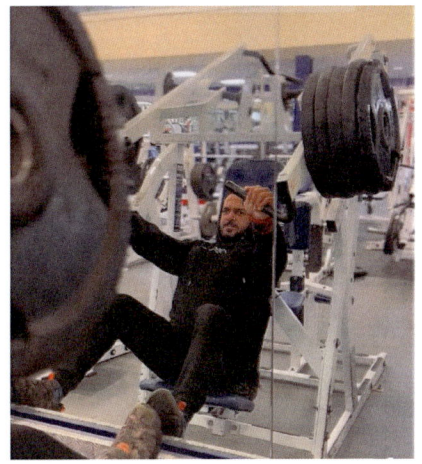

(Community & Camaraderie)

These unsung heroes roam the weight room, their eyes sharp, their protein shakes frothy, and their tank tops tighter than a clingy ex. Picture this, I just attempted a bench press, and the over enthusiastic spotter, fuelled by pre work out and dreams of glory dives in like a super hero. "I GOT YOU, BRO!" he screams, lifting the barbell with the strength of ten gym bros.

If I ever start before my spotter says 1,2,3 , I always get a comment "Mate, I was just adjusting my wrist wraps, you're not lifting weights, you're lifting dreams, so hold up." Haha.

Which is true indeed, every rep you take, you're building a dream physique sculpted in your mind.

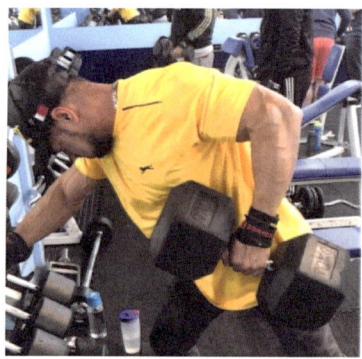

And so, dear friends, next time you spot a spotter, give them a nod of appreciation. They're the unsung heroes who prevent bench-press disasters, provide unintentional comedy, and keep the gym ecosystem in balance.

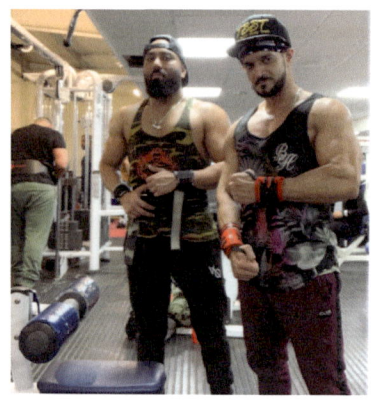
Sunday session with Fuzzy

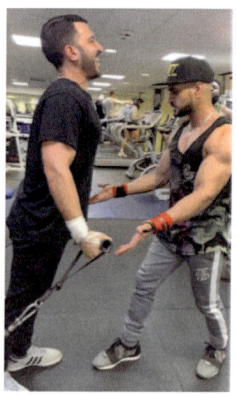
Bicep session with Gurch

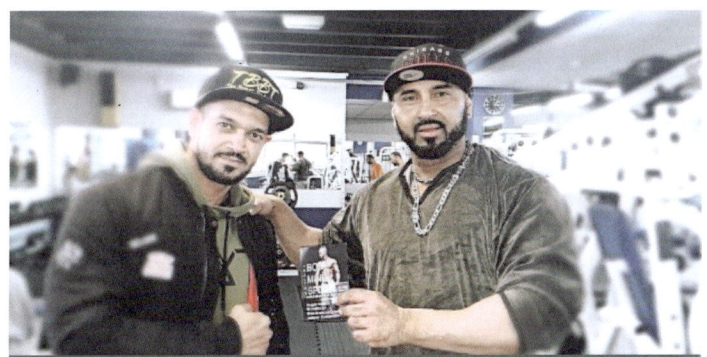

With Jay the fitness Guru

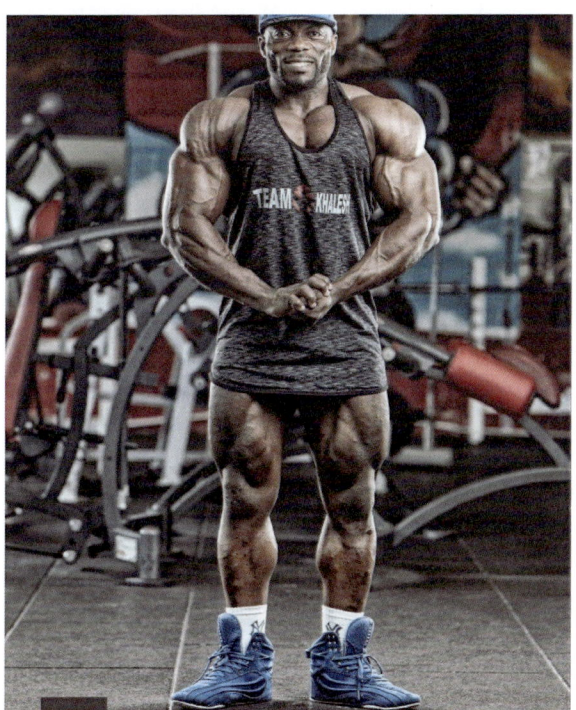

The Champ Michael, (Khalesh Trainer)

Remember: Behind every successful lift, there's a spotter thinking, "I hope they wipe down that bench afterward." haha

Chapter 18
The Blue Gym of Superheroes.

The big blue gym (Olympian Fitness) is a renowned fitness centre located in Hayes, Middlesex. Olympian Fitness offers a comprehensive range of facilities for both men and women. The gym boasts a mix of classic and modern equipment, ensuring that members have everything they need to achieve their fitness goals. Whether you're a seasoned athlete or a beginner, the friendly staff and inclusive environment make it an ideal place to work out. Olympian Fitness is more than just a gym; it's a hub where fitness enthusiasts come together, support each other, and prioritize overall well-being.

"Bonds forged in Iron".

In the Blue gym, where the clatter of weights and the rhythmic hum of treadmills created a symphony of determination, I found my tribe. We were a motley crew—each with our unique fitness goals—but bound by a shared passion for sweat, sore muscles, and the pursuit of strength.

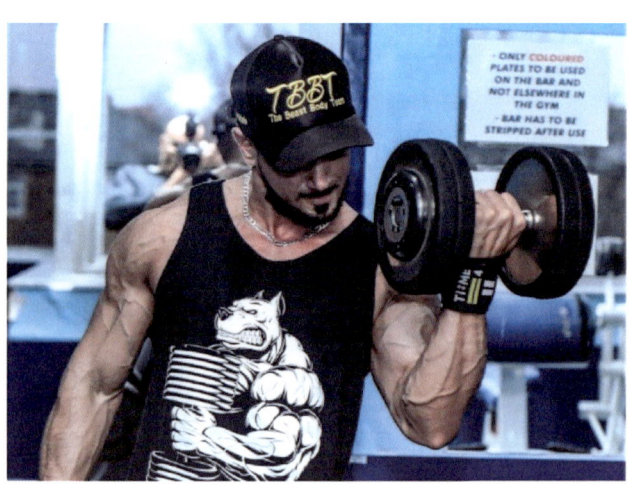

The Weightlifting Wizards - Ah, the weightlifting crew—the ones who grunted, strained, and occasionally dropped dumbbells with a resounding thud. Among them were Jai, Fuzzy, Max, Raheel, Harris, Tipu and many more who were fitness engineers by day and deadlift enthusiasts by night. Our friendship was forged in iron plates.

And so, within those mirrored walls and rubber-scented air, I discovered more than just physical strength. I found a tribe—a constellation of souls who lifted me higher than any dumbbell ever could. These people are not just gym buddies, but they are confidantes, and witnesses to each other's transformations.

So, the next time you step into your gym, look beyond the barbells and ellipticals. Seek out those kindred spirits—the ones who share your sweat, your dreams, and your protein shake recipes. Because sometimes, the best friendships are sculpted from iron and fuelled by endorphins.

In the next few pages, you will get to see some of these superheroes flexing their muscles, and posing and sharing their knowledge with you, and how they have transformed themselves into a fitness dynamo.

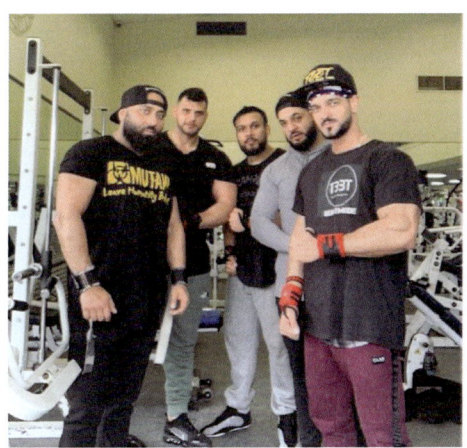
With Fuzzy, James, T and Raheel

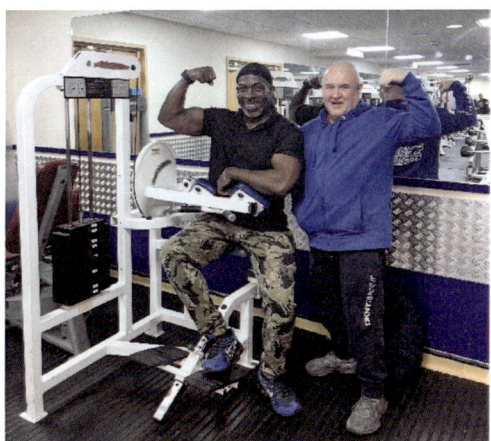
Alfred and Tony

The Blue Gym of Superheroes.

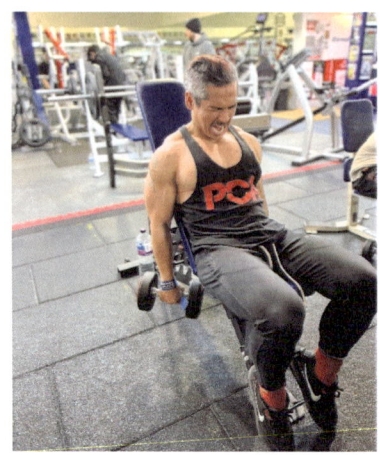
Max doing what he is best at.

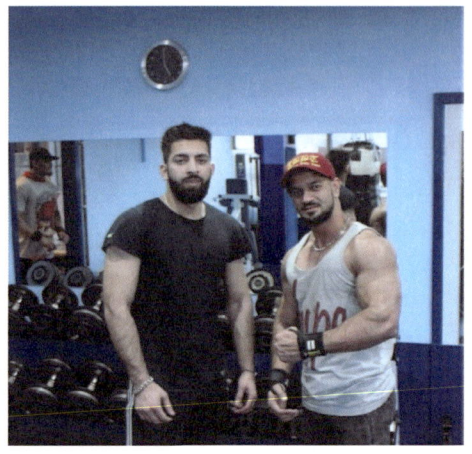
Everyday is training day for Imtiyaz

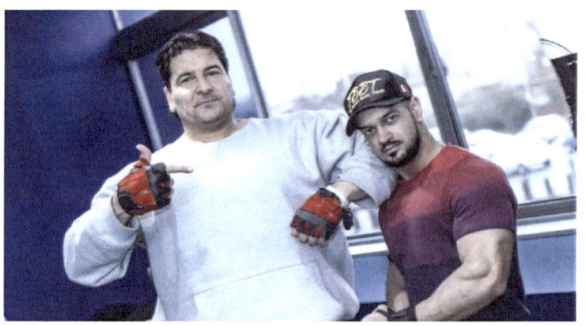
With the 7 Foot, Big Friendly Giant Javed

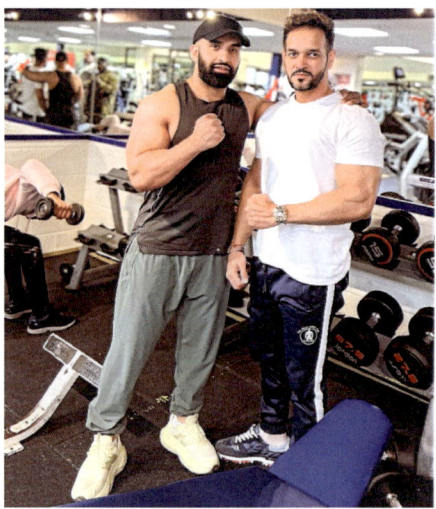
With Champ Ali

Let's explore some remarkable athletes, bodybuilders and Friends I have met, there are too many to list them all in this book. Here are a few who have been supportive. Whether they are flexing at the gym or grilling chicken breasts, this crew radiates power and dedication.

Firstly, I would like to introduce you to my Coach, this is the man who got me on stage to compete in Men's Physique and helped me start my fitness journey, My Coach, My Mentor in Fitness, who gave me the inspiration to get into the gym and transform my body into a fitness dynamo.

The support and motivation I have received from Omar has been top notch. There were days when I would struggle to reach my goals, but this man pushed me so hard, not just as his client, but pushed me like his own brother and made sure that I was able to achieve my goals. Indeed, it was a long process, and not easy. His knowledge in fitness took me to another level. I gained a lot of knowledge from Omar. I have been proud on all his achievements, there are certain people who you look up to, and Omar is one of them. I had the honour to feature Omar in my book and below is what he had to say about his experiences being a Pro card holder in Men's Physique and a successful Coach and a mentor.

Omar Ahmed (Coach)

Can you describe your experience in developing personalized fitness programs?

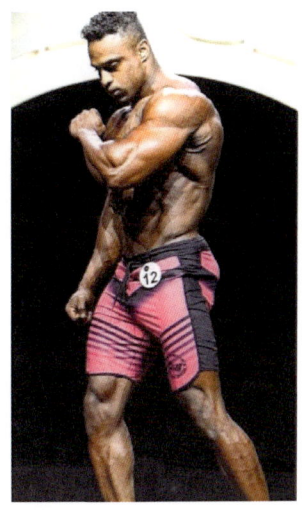

- I know Everyone is unique, because of their uniqueness, I develop a personalised plan for my clients, every client has a different body and goals to achieve, so each individual needs a plan according to their body, and I make sure I review their plans every week, and according to the results achieved I tweak them every week. I believe a plan should never be fixed, a plan should always change every week, according to the results of the client.

How do you assess the fitness level and needs of a new client?

- When it comes to new clients, its usually word of mouth because of the great work I have achieved with my previous clients, it's always a referral and recommendation in fitness industry. When I speak to new clients, I explain my process and how I work, and then leave it in the client's hands to decide if I am the right coach for them, because I believe that you are the one who decides who is the right coach for you. I present my vision to them and take it from there. 9 out of 10 are usually happy to proceed.

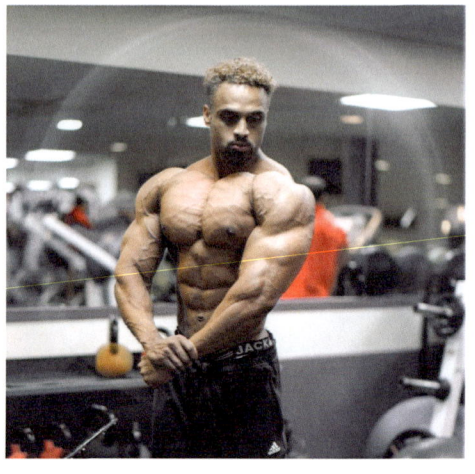

What inspired you to become a fitness coach?

- Well, I love helping people and love seeing them progress in their fitness journey, helping them achieve their goals and better themselves. Making them achieve their goals in the most effective and healthiest way possible. Their goal becomes my goal. It gives me pleasure when they transform their body, it is an achievement for them as well as me.

What do you think sets you apart from other fitness coaches?

- I feel more connected with my clients. I have a personal touch with them where they almost become a part of my family, they feel free to speak to me about anything, especially when they mess up in their diet. I am not really a coach who would make them feel uncomfortable, I like to have a open conversation with my clients, because some of them have personal problems that they might be going through, I try and help them through their process. I am connected to my clients more than other coaches A, B, C. It is a team process.

Have you ever been frustrated with your clients?

- Yes! I do sometimes, what I don't like is when my clients fail to do a weekly routine check up on their body with me. Because that way

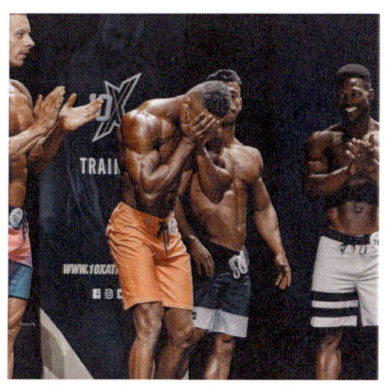

I come to know if they cheated on their meals and have not done what I have asked them to do. Being a Coach updates are very important, I give them time to get back to me, and set them straight back on the plan. Communication is vital as a Coach when you work as a team. It also happens when clients give excuses, it's too hard or I can't do it. I come in as a motivator and invest my time in them. If you really want to achieve your goals, you can, and nothing can stop you from reaching your goals. It depends how bad you want it.

How does it feel since you became a Pro Card Holder in Men's Physique?

- It feels amazing, because it took me years to achieve it and become into a fitness Dynamo, A Pro card holder, it didn't come easy, I struggled a lot to achieve this. Some people get Pro cards in 1 or 2 shows, I was one of the people who worked very hard to achieve it, that is why I value it the most. It raised my status in the fitness industry, I am more recognised amongst the athletes. The Coaches and Judges know me as a Fitness Public figure now. It is the experience that counts.

Do you look at things differently since you got your Pro Card?

- Definitely, Yes! Because I am at a pro level now, there is a big difference between an amateur show and a pro show. Now when it comes to prepare my clients and if he is an amateur, I prepare him according to the amateur show, and if he is going for a pro show then I prepare him or her according to the pro show, because for A Amateur show they

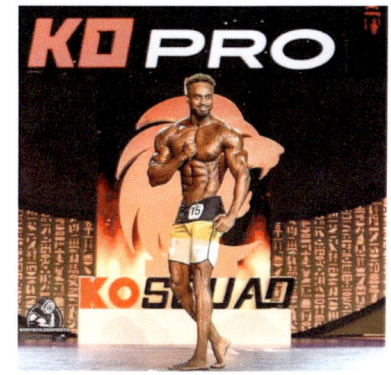

expect certain things, and for a Pro show they expect certain other things. The experience that I had personally by going from a amateur show to a pro show, and I had many different coaches in my journey, so it has taught me a lot of things and made me look at things differently.

What advice would you give youngsters who are just beginning their fitness journey?

- Be consistent and disciplined, whatever plan you have or the journey you are taking in fitness, be consistent. Listen to your coach, or get a coach, don't go around asking people, or you will get confused, you will get all sorts of different information which will make you wonder what is right and what is wrong.The most important thing is enjoying the process, because if you don't enjoy the process, you will end up quitting. Fitness journey is like a job. Be patient, things take time, gaining muscle takes time, there is no such thing as overnight body.

What is your vision and goal as a Fitness coach?

- I would like to create a team of Family and would like to have a camaraderie where I have 3 or 4 coaches under me, and inspire them to turn more athletes into Pro's, and qualify them into Olympia. Transform more amateur athletes into Pro's.

What would give you a greater joy to achieve goals as a Coach and Mentor?

- The joy of seeing someone else's achieve their goals, specially making someone get a Pro card, gives me more satisfaction then myself getting a Pro card, and I have felt this many times with my clients, especially when my clients have won the competition, or be it for from being a couch potato to getting 6 packs, the joy you see in your clients cannot be described in words.

Instagram: Omarahmed9

Jahangir: (Jai)

Jay is a force to be reckoned with, on the bodybuilding stage. Standing at 5'11" and weighing around 200 lbs, he boasts a massive frame that lives up to his nickname Jay. Keep an eye on him; he's still someone to watch for in 2024 in Men's Physique. His social media channels are filled with valuable tips and insights for fellow fitness enthusiasts. Jay as an athlete not only inspires us all but also exemplifies dedication, hard work, and passion in his pursuit of excellence. Whether you're a seasoned lifter or just starting out, following his journey can provide motivation and valuable insights for your own fitness goals. Below is what Jay had to say.

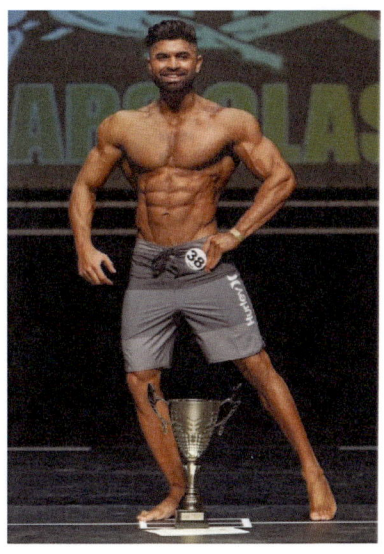

Describe your fitness journey?

Initially I had no intention to get on stage, I was a very athletic and sports driven person, used to be mainly in Athletics, in 2017 I ruptured my Achilles tendon, and the doctor said it was not possible for me to run again, but because of my competitive nature, I decided to move on to something else and it was the gym, Me still being on crutches, I had to transform my life into something I had never achieved before, and the best thing for me to do was to get in to bodybuilding, and since then the journey has carried on, and I never looked back.

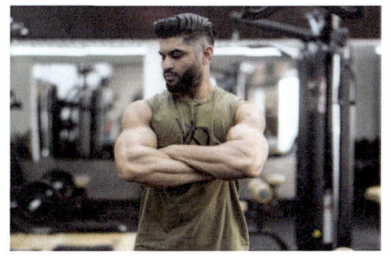

What is your biggest motivation and why?

Winning! Being an athlete since I was a kid, I have always excelled in physical activities, so I had the winner mentality in me. Coming second on a podium was not an option for me. My motivation is to excel and see myself at the top in bodybuilding.

What inspired you to become a fitness Dynamo?

I was heavily into Hollywood movies, my biggest inspiration was from the movie Commando featuring Arnold Schwarzenegger, just by looking at his physique I was motivated and inspired to take my journey on to the next level.

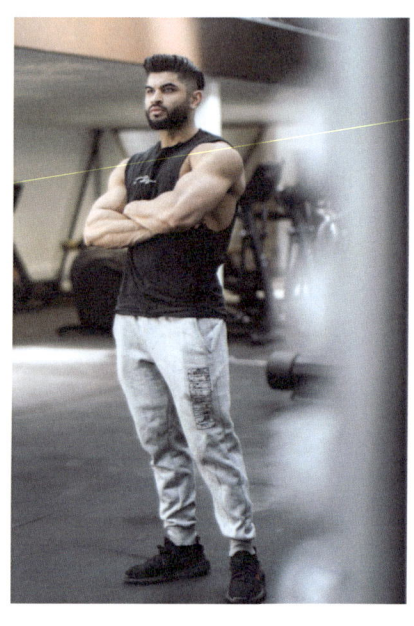

What made you become a fitness coach?

This will be an inspirational story for me to describe it to the readers, So I was given a placement from my college, I had 2 options, either join WH Smith or look for a placement outside for myself, and I chose Fitness First. I went 5 times to Fitness First, and out of the 5 times I was rejected 4 times. But the 5th time the fitness manager gave me a chance. I asked him to put me in there without any pay and

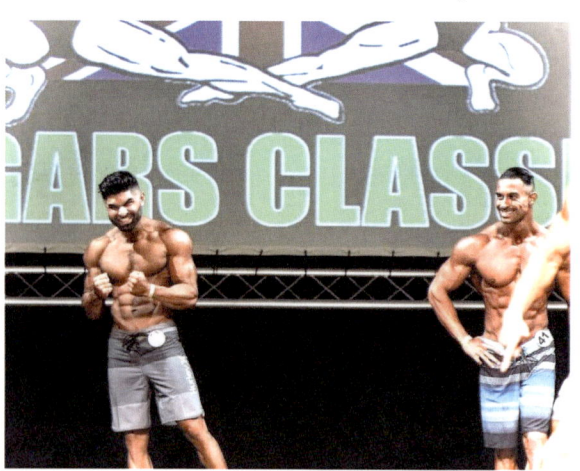

to prove myself, I was only 16, I excelled so good as a happy kid and learnt a lot from my fitness manager. He was so impressed by my work and fitness that he decided to send me on a Fitness Level 2 course as a fitness trainer. This is where my remarkable journey came into existence.

Do you have any plans of getting on stage soon?

Yes! The journey of being on stage is still unfinished, goal is to achieve my pro card and get on to the Olympia stage. So yes, there will be many more competitions to come.

How do you feel when you stand on stage competing with some Amazing competitors?

I prefer to be challenged by the best on stage, I want my victory to be hard earned, not easily given to me in my hands, I work hard, and my hard work pays off. Nothing comes easy, you must put long hours into fitness to achieve something great, you have to challenge yourself.

What would you advice our readers to follow in fitness?

Be very clear on your goals, your competition is only the previous you. You need to focus on being the best version of you, and not just follow the social media looks. The most important thing is the consistency with your diet and your programme, stay true to your plan and yourself and trust the process.

Do you have a mentor in fitness?

My first Mentor and coach was Michael (Khalesh Trainer) He is the one who got me started, He helped me and guided me on my first few shoes, he is the one who made me fall in love with bodybuilding, also not to forget my older brother Akmal who first got me in the gym and motivated me to lift weights. I also learn from my fellow friends in the gym, who are fitness dynamos themselves, like Harris, Saheeb, Omar.

What is your vision in fitness?

I have 2 visions in fitness, one is a Personal Vision of representing the best version of myself on Olympia stage. My other vision is to open my own gym and help people achieve their goals. Impact their lifestyle and make them achieve their goals.

Instagram: jkfitness.pt

Iwona Michalska: (Evee)

In a world where gender stereotypes persist, Evee stands out as a trailblazer. As a female Athlete, she has defied societal expectations, shattered stereotypes, and carved her own path to success. With unwavering determination and a relentless pursuit of her passion, Evee has become an inspiration for women who dare to challenge conventions. Her sculpted physique, dedication to training, and unwavering spirit serve as a testament to the power of resilience and the pursuit of excellence. Let's delve into the remarkable journey of this modern-day woman who lifts not only weights but also barriers.

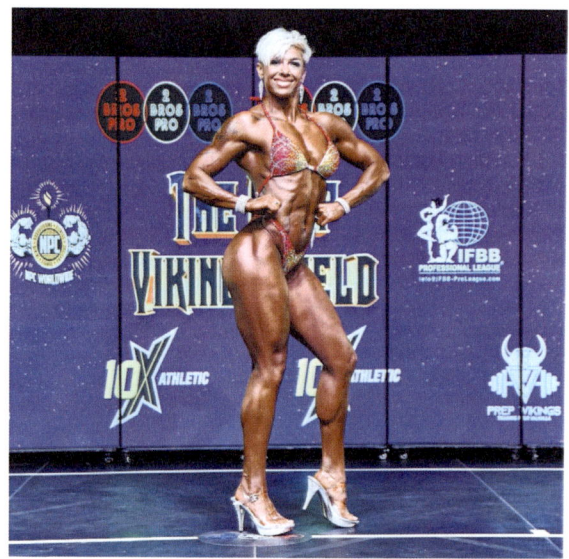

How has your fitness journey been so far?

What an experience my fitness journey has been, I started my bodybuilding at the end of 2019, when my friend introduced me to free weights. I still remember lifting the first barbell with weights, I couldn't believe how it changed my body time after time I lifted weights. The feeling itself was so amazing, and the joy it gave me mentally. And as days passed, I wanted to look better, I am very thankful to my first coach and Friend Stefano to push me to achieve my goals.

What inspired you to become a Fitness dynamo?

I was inspired by Arnold Schwarzenegger, I used to watch all his videos, and documentaries, which helped me in self-development and knowledge of fitness. As we all remember, unfortunately we went into lockdown, meaning our second home, our gym was about to shut down for a while. But that didn't stop me, I collected weight plates, barbells, dumbbell's and started training at home. Over those 6 months I gained great amount of muscle mass, So, my mind was ready for more challenges.

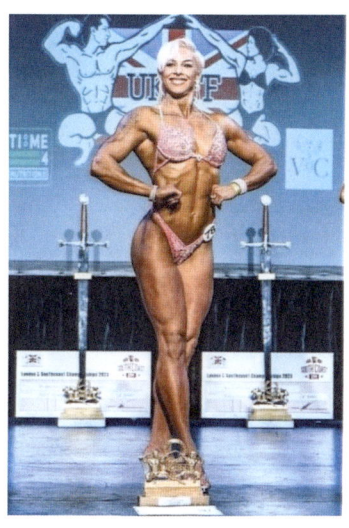

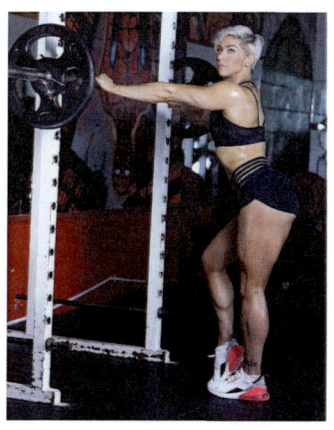

When did you decide to get on stage and compete?

I have some great athletes in my gym who inspired me to get on stage, with the help of my Coach-Michael (Khalesh Trainer), he helped me prep for my first bodybuilding show in figure division in November 2021, I started preparing for this show in the mid-July 2021. Since then, I have been competing nonstop to achieve better results.

How do you feel after achieving your Pro Card?

I feel amazing after achieving my Pro Card, I got my pro card with GBO in June 2022. The Joy is unbelievable, after receiving my Pro card I have been more serious and dedicated towards fitness. Now my dream is to take this to another level and stand on Olympia stage and bring the trophy back home.

Did bodybuilding change your life? How do you change other people's life by being a coach?

Yes! Body building changed my life completely, and I wanted to change others through my achievements. So, between being a mum and working part time, I became A certified Personal Trainer and Nutritionist. I help people by making them reach their goals, some are struggling to lose weight, while other struggling to put muscle size. I make sure I help all my clients, no matter what their journey is.

What advice would you give to the young generation?

My advice would be, join the gym, make it a habit, eat good, don't cheat on your meals. Dedicate your time to the gym, the results you see will be amazing. It takes time to achieve your fitness goals, stick to it and you will see the results flow.

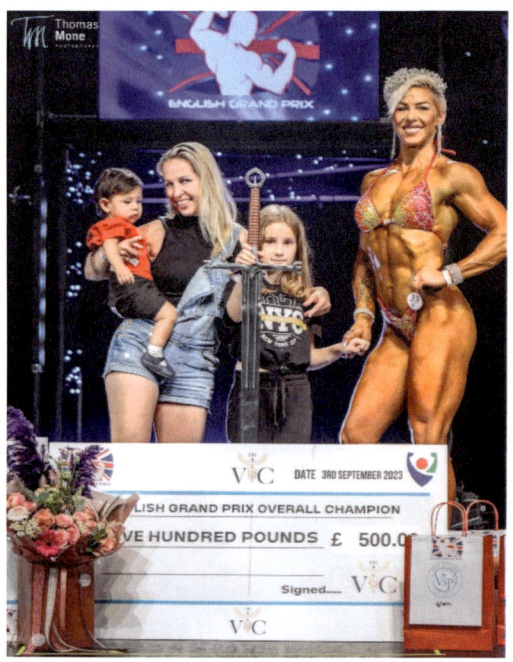

Instagram : train_with_evee_pt

Harris Mehboob

Meet Harris, a man whose life revolves around iron, sweat, and the relentless pursuit of physical excellence. As a certified personal trainer and the proud owner of **Anytime Fitness Gym**, Harris embodies the fusion of passion and profession. His journey began with a humble set of dumbbells in the gym as a beginner, but over the years, it transformed into a thriving fitness empire.

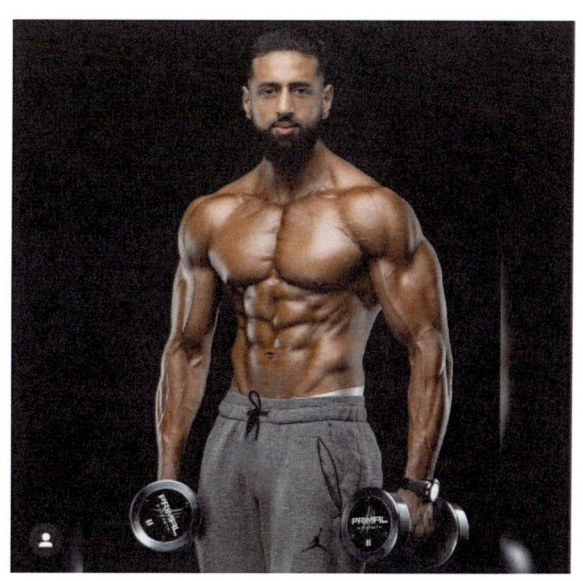

Describe your fitness journey to our readers?

I want to share my fitness journey and how it has changed me as a person. Sure, I've had ups & downs. I've gained, I've lost, and I've learnt. Everyone's journey is different, and this one is mine.

Fitness is not about being better than anyone else. It's about being better than you used to be. I've always been passionate about fitness and working out from a very young age but decided to take it seriously when I started my university back in 2011. Initially when I started, I didn't know the technicality behind the workout routine. I had no idea what to do in the gym, nor where to even begin, but as time went on, I started doing my research. I had few friends who were already going to the gym, and they really helped me out to work around gym equipment, machines. Then I decided to make a change in my fitness routine and do my Level 2 & Level 3 qualification to pursue my fitness journey further.

What inspired you to become a Fitness Coach?

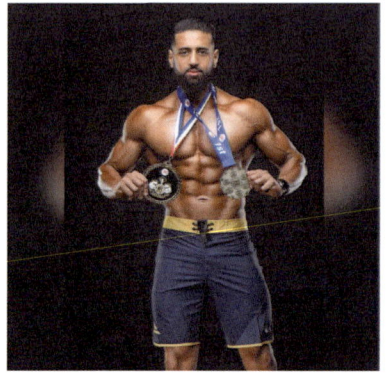

I wanted to help people, and learn more about Fitness, I had to learn how to transform my body, So I decided to get myself qualified by doing Level 2 & level 3 qualification in fitness. I started to understand my body better and adapt to things that could really help me with my fitness goals. A lot of my friends started asking me for advice and if I could help them with their fitness journey, my answer was, Yes! This is how it all started being a Coach to my friends and my clients.

What made you get on stage and compete?

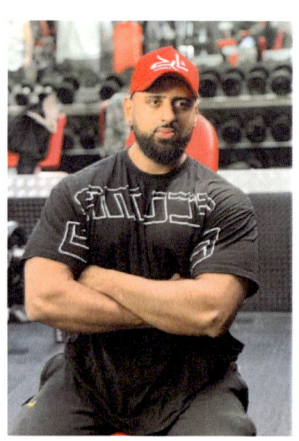

To push myself even further I decided to do and compete in different federations. I still remember My first ever show was back in 2019, I had all my friends and clients coming to that show and I won in my first ever show, that was just the start. I was so proud that I managed to prove myself and all the hard work for the prep I did, paid off.

Since then, I never looked back I've done a lot more shows now with different federations like 2bros.

How was your experience as a Men's physique champion in UKBFF and further going on to 2 Bros?

My experience with both these federations was amazing, it taught me a lot as an Athlete, the other athletes I competed with were in amazing shape, and that was my motivation of becoming better and better each time I stepped on stage. You learn from your competitions.

Do you have your own Gym?

Yes! Now I own my own gym called Anytime Fitness in St.Paul's Cathedral Central London. It was a dream come true. I always dreamt as a kid that one day I will have my own gym, nothing is impossible if you have a Vision. Your dream could be unrealistic for your friends or other people, but if you believe in this vision, you will make it to the top. Never give up.

How long did you take to become a successful Coach and Mentor?

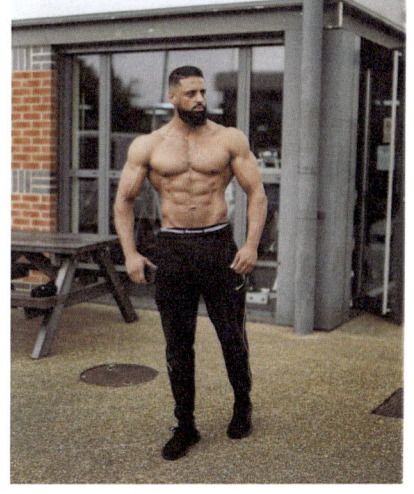

I would say every step is a learning curve for me, it took me years to come to this level, and I still have a lot to learn. I learn from my juniors too and vice versa. I help my clients to achieve their goals, I want to be the best coach ever. I have many clients on my list who are stepping on stage and are winning the competitions. I would like to continue my journey and help more people to change their lives.

So, next time you step into Anytime Core Fitness, look for the man with calloused hands and a perpetual smile. That's Harris—the architect of dreams, the curator of sweat-soaked stories, and the embodiment of what it means to **live strong**.

Instagram: Teamharis.pt

Maximo Edralin: (Max)

The spotlight awaits. Let me introduce you to the epitome of men's physique mastery (Max), the embodiment of discipline, and the living canvas of sculpted artistry. His passion for fitness ignites like a spark, fuelled by iron plates and unwavering determination. From the very first bicep curl, Max knew he was destined for greatness.

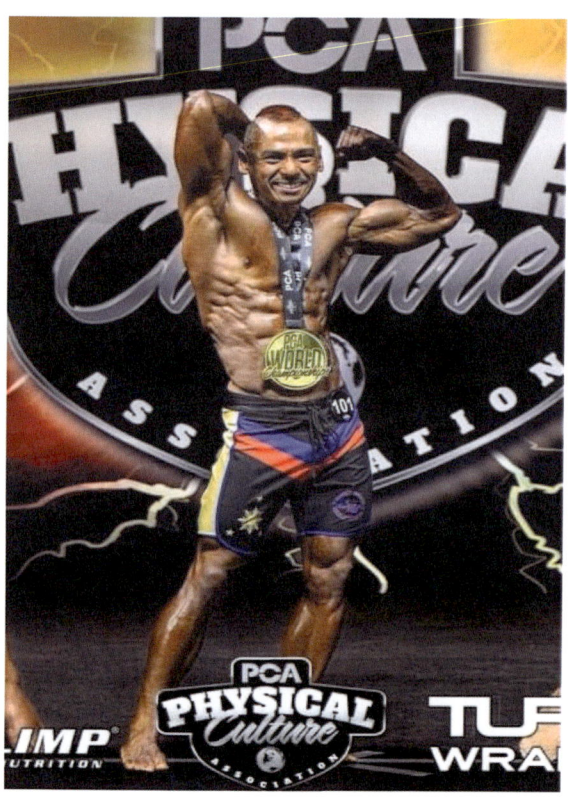

Tell us something about your fitness journey?

I've been resistance training since I was 13 years old! The 32-year journey has had many goals, lessons and sports involved, including football, wing chun, boxing, callisthenics and obstacle course racing. Men's physique bodybuilding has only been part of my life for the last 8 years.

What is your biggest motivation?

I think being a small/short guy I've always been motivated to physically be able to stand out among the tallest/biggest guys and I also like to prove I can build optimal muscle whilst being 100% natural! Bettering myself within my own limits has always been my motivation. Of course, I've had many sporting heroes and icons, but I've never tried to be "like" them or do things like them, although, I was always inspired by their abilities and work ethic!

What inspired you to become a fitness Dynamo?

I think after many years of training and physique competing self-coached, I have been known to many around me (in all environments) 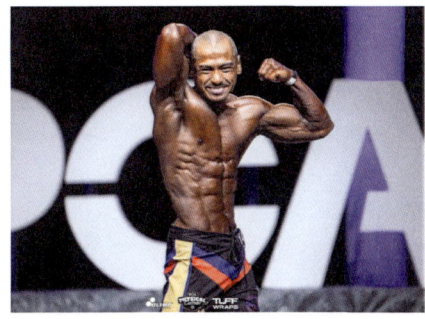 as the man who knows a lot about building muscle and reducing body fat. So, I love to learn about different training techniques, how new science research affects the way we train, and how to maximise training. With this knowledge I'm inspired to improve the thinking and knowledge of others as much as possible. The desire to learn from myself is something I also find very inspirational; their energy gives me more energy in the industry.

Do you enjoy being a fitness coach?

I really do! I think helping people achieve their fitness goals is very rewarding and the challenges inspires me to learn more!

How do you feel after becoming a world champion?

Of course, I am very happy about it. But it's also a relief achieving such an

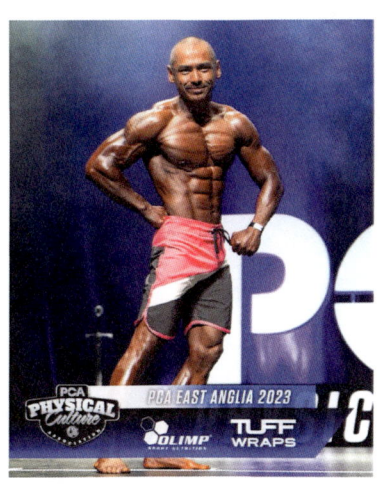

award after many years of pushing at a demanding and subjective sport!

What would you advise our readers if they want to become a fitness Champ like you?

You must enjoy the journey, know that there is not one way to achieve such a goal and creating a lifestyle and mindset is the best way to move onward and upward!

Do you have a mentor in fitness?

Growing up during my 32-year fitness journey I've had a few mentors and people to inspire me. Now as a mature, knowledgeable trainer I have a handful of people that I follow online for new information, but it's good practice to read up about any techniques or methods that are new, or even old!

Do you encourage young kids to join gym?

I do, obviously with good guidance. They also need to stay within a particular level of intensity and make sure technique & form is very good! I have 2 young boys of my own that I encourage to train whether with load, bodyweight, or even when conditioning for a particular sport.

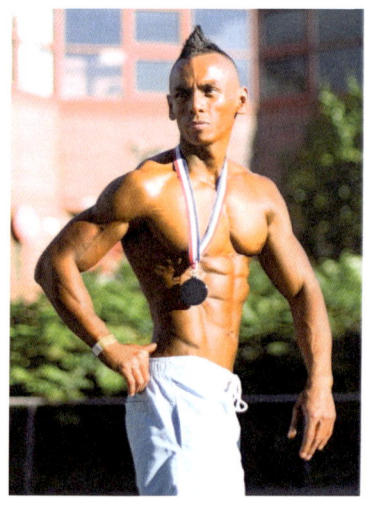

What do you enjoy the most in being a world champion?

Knowing I have the credentials to add to my knowledge. Too many people only listen to the elite athletes online or the genetically blessed (that isn't always obvious). The most knowledgeable people are often those who had to think outside the box and work differently to achieve in areas they are weakest or struggled with.

Instagram: Maximum_edralin_pt

Finally, I thought I should write a bit about myself or maybe a poem to describe my fitness journey, and how I got on stage and what made me push it beyond the limits. Surrounded by the rhythmic clank of iron plates and the scent of determination, I discovered my passion for bodybuilding. Little did I know that this sweaty sanctuary would become the stage for my metamorphosis—a transformation not only of muscle but of mind and spirit. My journey began with a single dumbbell, as it does for most of us, a modest weight that felt like Atlas burden at the time. I was an eager novice, fuelled by visions of sculpted physiques and the allure of standing under the spotlight.

Building the foundation was not easy, I quickly realized that bodybuilding wasn't just about lifting weights; it was an intricate dance between science and art. I devoured knowledge like a ravenous beast, studying nutrition, biomechanics, and the delicate balance of macros. Each rep became a step toward mastery, and every meal a brushstroke on the canvas of my physique.

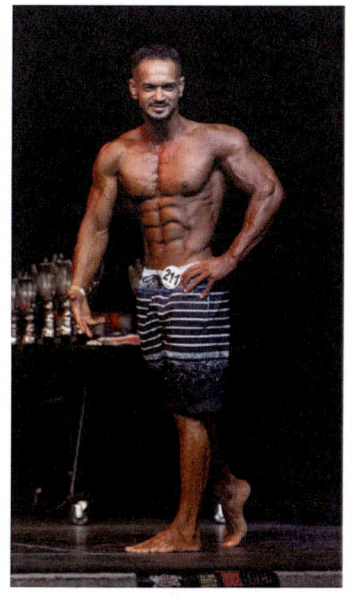

The Mental battle, As the months turned into years, I faced mental hurdles as formidable as any squat rack. Doubt whispered in my ear during gruelling pre-dawn workouts, questioning my resolve. But I silenced it with determination, the same determination that would propel me onto the stage.

This is where the spotlight beckons, my first ever Men's Physique competition in July 2018, finally, the day arrived, the culmination of countless early mornings, sore muscles, and chicken breasts. Under the unforgiving glare of the stage lights, I flexed, posed, and bared my soul. The judges scrutinized every striation, every curve, and every bead of sweat. But I wasn't merely showcasing my physique; I was sharing my journey, a testament to human potential. I had some amazing athletes standing on stage with me, I was nervous about my Posing, my smile, everything was a question and doubt in my mind, but that didn't stop me, it was one of the best experiences of my life, since then I never stopped, I went on to do 10 more competitions after that. The hunger in me was growing, wanting to be the best. It was Me vs Me. My dream was to be the best of the best.

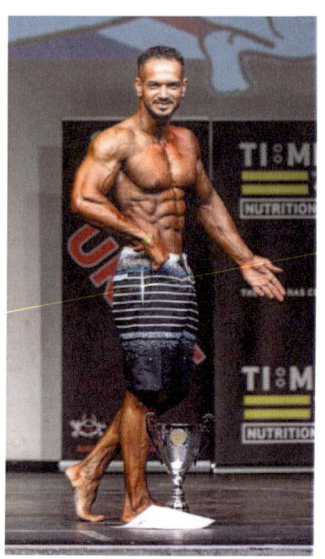

Beyond the tanning oil and the posing trunks, I have realized that bodybuilding is a gateway to wisdom. The pursuit of physical excellence had honed my mental fortitude. I devoured scientific journals, dissected training protocols, and delved into the psychology of peak performance. I became an athlete of knowledge—an ambassador for the symbiosis of body and brain.

I got so deep into fitness that I decided to make my own fitness brand "The Beast Body Team", and it became my Instagram name, it took no time for it to get noticed, when I started sharing my Fitness Journey, and then later on decided to get qualified as a Personal trainer and Nutritionist, which got me more involved in the gym and help and train people to achieve their goals. I became a mentor for my clients, it gave me satisfaction as I started to change their mindset and physique.

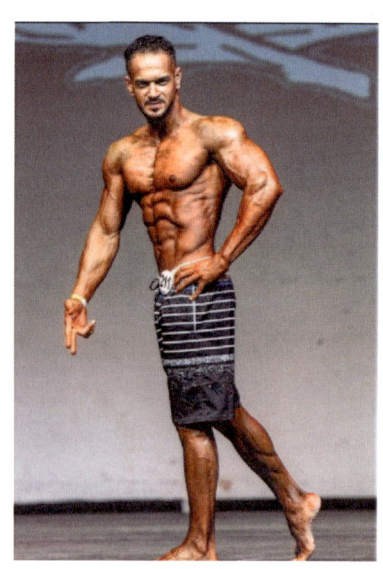

To have a well sculpted physique it takes time. My advice is never giving up on your dreams, and never give up on your body, if you have a vision, and you can see it, then for sure you can achieve it. There is no such thing as impossible. If it looks unrealistic to your friends and family, let it be! You are the one who can make it happen. So, stick to your unrealistic dreams my dear readers, and make them into reality.

So, here I stand, not just as an Athlete but as a seeker of truth—a lifter of weights and ideas. The stage is my canvas, and I painted it with my sweat, sacrifice, and sheer willpower. And as the curtain falls, I know that my journey has only just begun—a perpetual ascent towards the summit of mind, muscle, and motion.

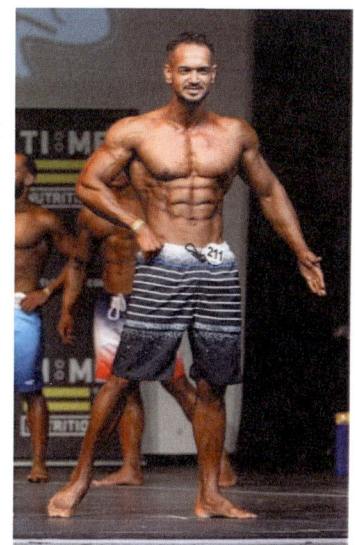

Instagram: thebeastbodyteam

Chapter 19

Should you have a personal Trainer or Mentor?

Having a **fitness mentor or coach** can significantly enhance your fitness journey. It helps you reach your fitness goals, especially a well-qualified trainer with good experience in nutrition and training can be helpful.

1. **Personalized Guidance:**
    - A mentor tailors their advice to your unique needs, goals, and limitations.
    - They provide personalized workout plans, nutrition guidance, and lifestyle recommendations.
    - Whether in person or virtually, they will keep you on track.

2. **Motivation and Accountability:**
    - A mentor keeps you motivated and accountable.
    - Knowing someone is tracking your progress encourages consistency and effort.

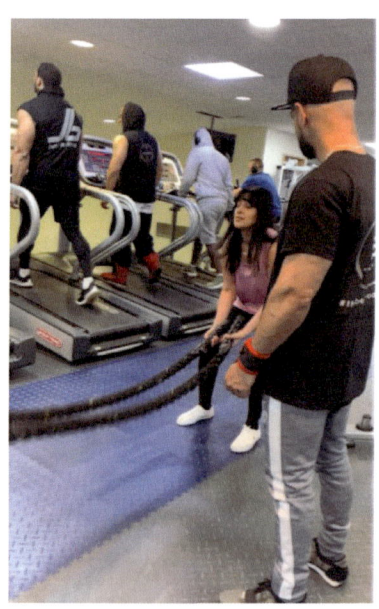

3. **Expertise and Experience:**
    - Fitness Mentors have extensive knowledge and experience.
    - Beyond workouts they impart valuable health and fitness information to help you maintain a healthy lifestyle.

- They guide you through proper form, exercise selection, and recovery strategies.

4. **Overcoming Plateaus:**
   - When progress stalls, a Personal trainer helps you break through plateaus.
   - They adjust your routines, introduce variety, and provide fresh perspectives.

5. **Emotional Support:**
   - Fitness journeys can be challenging. A mentor offers emotional support.
   - Trainer fosters positive mindset, banishing self-doubt and negativity.
   - They understand setbacks, celebrate victories, and keep you focused.

6. **Learning Opportunities:**
   - Personal trainers share insights, tips, and evidence-based practices.
   - You learn from their successes and mistakes.

Having a fitness trainer and mentor provides guidance, encouragement, and expertise. Whether you're a beginner or an experienced athlete, their support can elevate your fitness game!

Below is a good example of one of my many clients Sunny and how he transformed his body, with a strong mindset and dedication.

A Journey of Transformation

Meet **Sunny**, an extraordinary Project Manager who defied a sedentary lifestyle and embarked on a remarkable fitness journey. His struggle with weight began in his 20's, and working as a project manager only exacerbated it, leading to a staggering **92 kg**.

But Sunny decided to take charge of his health. With my guidance, he aligned himself with his fitness goals and committed to change.

The results were astounding, Sunny shed an incredible **12 kg**! Today, he stands as a testament to what determination and consistency can achieve.

Here's how he transformed from into a fitness dynamo:

1. **Mindset Shift**: Sunny recognized that his sedentary lifestyle was detrimental to his well-being. He made a conscious decision to prioritize fitness.
2. **Nutrition**: He revamped his eating habits, focusing on balanced meals, portion control, and nutrient-dense foods.
3. **Exercise**: He gradually incorporated physical activity into his routine. Whether it was brisk walking, jogging, or strength training, he stayed committed.
4. **Support System**: Having a coach and a supportive community made all the difference. We provided motivation, accountability, and expert guidance.
5. **Consistency**: Sunny didn't expect overnight results. He stayed consistent, celebrating small victories along the way.

Today, he is physically and emotionally fit, inspiring those around him to take their fitness seriously. Sunny's journey reminds us that transformation is possible, no matter where we start.

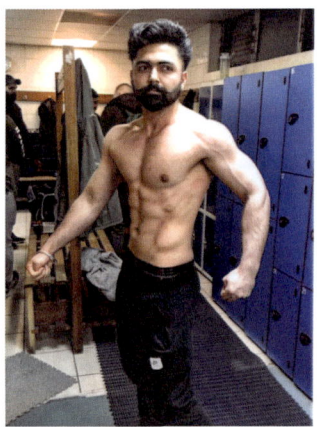

👏 **Congratulations, Sunny!** Your dedication and resilience are truly commendable. Keep shining as a fitness dynamo!

Chapter 20

The Finish Line and Beyond.

Embrace Your Fitness Journey.

Here's a concise and motivating conclusion of this book.

We've explored the dynamic world of fitness, delving into exercise routines, nutrition, and mental resilience. As you close these pages, remember that your journey towards a healthier, stronger you, is ongoing. Here are some key takeaways:

1. **Physical Health**: Regular physical activity isn't just about aesthetics; it's a powerful tool for enhancing your overall well-being. Engaging in exercise can reduce the risk of diseases, improve physical functioning, and boost your quality of life.

2. **Cognitive Performance**: Exercise isn't limited to the body; it also benefits the mind. As you lace up your sneakers, know that you're sharpening your cognitive abilities and enhancing mental clarity.

3. **Psychological Well-Being**: The gym isn't just a place for lifting weights; it's a sanctuary for stress relief. Whether it's a brisk jog or a yoga session, physical activity releases endorphins, lifting your mood and promoting mental balance.

4. **Consistency Matters**: Fitness isn't a sprint; it's a marathon. Embrace the small victories—the extra rep, the healthier meal choice, the commitment to daily movement. These consistent efforts compound over time, leading to lasting results.

5. **Community and Support**: Seek out like-minded individuals who share your fitness goals. Whether it's a workout buddy, an

online community, or a supportive coach, surround yourself with positivity and encouragement.

6. **Celebrate Progress**: Celebrate every milestone, no matter how small. Whether it's shedding a few pounds, mastering a new exercise, or simply feeling more energetic, acknowledge your progress and keep pushing forward.

Remember, your fitness journey is unique. Embrace the process, listen to your body, and stay committed. You're not just building a better physique; you're cultivating resilience, discipline, and a healthier life.

Lastly, Thank you for joining me on this adventure. Now go out there and conquer your fitness goals—one squat, one healthy meal, and one positive thought at a time!

Wishing you all the best in your Fitness Endeavours!

Mind, Muscle, & Motion

YOUR WEIGHTS ARE LIKE CHISEL AND YOU'RE THE SCULPTOR, ONE DAY IT WILL SCULPT YOUR BODY, THE WAY YOU IMAGINED IT.

SAHEEB DADAN

Acknowledgement

I extend my deepest gratitude to all the individual athletes and entities who have contributed to this book. Their unwavering support, encouragement and inspiration has been invaluable.

To my family and friends who stood by me in late nights and countless revisions, who provided laughter, encouragement, and the occasional reality check, your presence made this journey memorable. Thanks for all the advice, expertise and critical feedback which challenged me to grow as a writer. I dedicate this book also to my sisters Kudseya, Zuhaina and to my brother Ali who are sadly no longer with me, but always in my heart and memories.

Finally, to you, dear reader, for embarking on this literary adventure. May these words resonate with you, evoke emotions and linger in your thoughts long after you turn the last page.

A Beautiful postscript written by my friend Fuzzy.

PS : Captured in the heart of our fitness journey, this book embodies the spirit of determination and solidarity. Surrounded by friends, each of us pushing our limits and supporting one another, we've created a vibrant community driven by a shared passion for health and strength. From lifting weights to perfecting form, every bead of sweat and every smile tells a story of perseverance and joy. Together, we not only transform our bodies but also build unbreakable bonds, proving that the gym is more than just a place to train – it's where we grow stronger, together.

"Get ready for the highly anticipated release of book version 2, Arriving soon!"

www.ingramcontent.com/pod-product-compliance
Lightning Source LLC
Chambersburg PA
CBRC100215040426
42333CB00035B/71